Clinical Aspects
of Microdialysis

Edited by
A. Mendelowitsch, H. Langemann,
B. Alessandri, H. Landolt,
O. Gratzl

Acta Neurochirurgica
Supplement 67

SpringerWienNewYork

Dr. Aminadav Mendelowitsch
University Neurosurgical Clinic, Kantonsspital Basel, Basel, Switzerland

Dr. Helen Langemann
Department of Research, Kantonsspital Basel, Basel, Switzerland

Dr. Beat Alessandri
Department of Research, Kantonsspital Basel, Basel, Switzerland

Dr. Hans Landolt
Neurosurgical Clinic, Kantonsspital Aarau, Aarau, Switzerland

Professor Dr. Otmar Gratzl
University Neurosurgical Clinic, Kantonsspital Basel, Basel, Switzerland

Typesetting: Thomson Press, New Delhi, India

Graphic design: Ecke Bonk

Printed on acid-free and chlorine free bleached paper

With 56 Figures

Library of Congress Cataloging-in-Publication Data

Clinical aspects of microdialysis / edited by A. Mendelowitsch ... [et al.].
    p.   cm. -- (Acta neurochirurgica. Supplement ; 67)
   Based on the First International Meeting on Clinical Aspects of Microdialysis held in March 1995 in Basel, Switzerland.
   Includes bibliographical references and index.
   ISBN 3-211-82834-6 (alk. paper)
   1. Brain microdialysis--Congresses.   I. Mendelowitsch, A., 1957-
. II. International Meeting on Clinical Aspects of Microdialysis
(1st : 1995 : Basel, Switzerland) III. Series.
   [DNLM: 1. Brain Diseases--diagnosis--congresses.
2. Microdialysis--methods--congresses. 3. Brain--physiopathology-
-congresses. 4. Monitoring, Physiologic--methods--congresses.   W1
AC8661 no.67 1996 / WL 348 C641 1996]
RC386.6.B73C56 1996
616.8'04754--dc20
DNLM/DLC
for Library of Congress   96-18565
                                                                    CIP

ISSN 0065-1419
ISBN-13: 978-3-7091-7426-5   e-ISBN-13: 978-3-7091-6894-3
DOI: 10.1007/978-3-7091-6894-3

Preface

Microdialysis is a minimally invasive method which enables continuous monitoring of parameters in the extracellular space of various tissues. It has been investigated in animal models for over a decade, and many publications have provided insight into its advantages and disadvantages. However, in spite of its enormous potential for revealing metabolic processes in normal and pathological tissue, microdialysis in humans is still in its infancy.

Clinical neurointensive medicine nowadays demands much more than conventional monitoring methods. As already shown by jugular bulb measurements of oxygen and lactate, in the future clinicians will want to have access to continuous neurochemical information from the patient. This information could be used to prevent those enigmatic secondary lesions which play such a negative role in neurointensive medicine, or at least enable treatment of them at an early stage. The extensive information now available from the laboratory would help with the interpretation of clinical analogues.

In the University Clinic of Neurosurgery in Basel we have been involved in the field of microdialytic monitoring for several years and have recognised the problems, both technical and ethical, which are involved in taking the difficult step from animal experiments to clinical application. In 1994 we thought that research on clinical microdialysis had reached the stage which would enable scientists and clinicians to have many fruitful discussions. We therefore decided to organise the First International Meeting on Clinical Aspects of Microdialysis in our city in March 1995. The response from participants all over the world was highly encouraging.

This volume includes some of the contributions given at the Meeting. About a third of the presentations were concerned with basic aspects, and were thus very valuable especially for the clinicians in the audience. The rest dealt with the most recent clinical aspects and covered a wide range of subjects – for instance cerebral monitoring in critical care patients and during operations, new designs for probes and for on-line monitoring, measurements in blood, etc. The whole spectrum of present-day applications can be studied.

Final discussions at the Meeting showed that there are two main problems involved in the clinical use of microdialysis. First, patients are not inbred experimental animals, and their brains are usually in an extremely pathological and unstable condition, so the measured levels of parameters in their dialysates (even in those from relatively undamaged tissue) are extremely variable. Some of this variability can be attributed to differences in the conditions of microdialysis, for instance in relative recovery, and it was suggested that these might be standardised. Second, for a monitoring system to be clinically relevant, parameters must be found which have predictive value for pathological events such as secondary ischaemia in head trauma patients. There were encouraging indications at the Meeting that such paramaters do in fact exist. However, before these two problems can be finally solved, a large data bank must be built up; thus cooperation between the various groups working in the field is essential. This is our common task for the future.

We are confident that there will soon be widespread use of microdialysis in the clinic, not only for cerebral monitoring (the aspect of major interest to readers of Acta Neurochirurgica), but also for other applications, some of which were presented at the Meeting (neonatal monitoring in adipose tissue, muscle monitoring, control of drug levels in patients, glucose monitoring in diabetics). We also hope this volume will succeed in arousing interest in this fascinating method, which is able to tell us bedside what is going on in the patient's brain at the molecular level.

The Editors

Contents

Listed in Current Contents

Acta Neurochir (1996) [Suppl] 67: 1–5

Possible Glial Contribution of Rat Hippocampus Lactate as Assessed with Microdialysis and Stress

O. Elekes[1,*], K. Venema[2], F. Postema[2], R. Dringen[2], B. Hamprecht[2], and J. Korf[1]

[1]Department of Biological Psychiatry, Groningen University, The Netherlands and [2]Physiologisch-chemisches Institut, Universität Tübingen, Federal Republic of Germany

Summary

Microdialysis for the continuous monitoring of lactate ("lactography") was applied in rat brain hippocampus in an attempt to establish whether lactate is of neuronal or glial origin. Lactate was analyzed with an electrochemical assay after enzymatic oxidation in dialysates derived from a short-term (1 or 2 days after implantation of the probe) and a long-term (14 or 15 days) preparation. In the short-term experiment the lactate levels in the dialysate were higher without glucose in the perfusate, whereas in the long-term experiment a several fold increase in lactate was observed in the presence of 5 mM glucose. During stress, increases in lactate were virtually similar both in the acute (with or without glucose in the perfusate) and in the chronic preparation (response in the presence of glucose only). In the long term preparation presence of reactive astroglia cells was visualized immunohistochemically with antibodies against glial fibrillary acidic protein. Damage of the hippocampus and the corpus callosum was seen in the chronic preparation with silver impregnation staining. These results emphasize the importance of the presence of glucose in the perfusate and they are consistent with the idea that glial cells contribute to extracellular lactate in the rat hippocampus in vivo and that stress activates the astroglial glycogen pool.

Keywords: Astroglia; lactate; microdialysis; stress.

Abbreviations: GFAP = glial fibrillary acidic protein.

Introduction

Using microdialysis extracellular lactate derived from various brain regions can be monitored ('lactography') with on- and off-line detection techniques [9, 10, 11, 17, 24]. Either technique of lactography shows that extracellular levels of lactate are easily altered under physiological and pathological conditions. So,

for instance, electro-convulsive shock, mild stress and several drugs affect the concentration of extracellular lactate in the rat hippocampus [1, 2, 5, 6, 7, 13].

The major source or sources of extracellular lactate has thus far not been established. A variety of experiments has demonstrated the virtually exclusive cerebral origin of extracellular lactate [10, 13, 15]. Such experiments can, however, not prove whether lactate is derived from a glial or neuronal metabolic pool. In the hippocampus glycogen phosphorylase was virtually exclusively confined to astroglial cells [20]. When glycogen is degraded, lactate, rather than glucose leaves the astroglial cell [3, 4, 26] and may then serve as an energy substrate in surrounding neurons [19, 22]. If lactate is derived from glial glycogen, lactate synthesis and efflux is expected to be affected when glucose is infused via the dialysis probe. When, however, glucose in the tissue around the probe is exclusively derived from the circulation, little if any effect of glucose added to or removed from the perfusate is to be expected. Glucose dependency would thus be stronger when the dialysis probe is maintained in situ for a period of 2 weeks, when glial cells have proliferated. Glial response is anticipated either as the result of damage due to the placement of the probe, to subsequent neuronal degeneration or to both [8, 23].

Baseline levels of lactate and lactate levels after exposure to immobilization stress were determined in the absence or presence of glucose in the perfusion medium. The astroglyosis was shown immunohistochemically by staining for glial fibrillary acidic protein (GFAP), and damage was shown with a silver impregnation staining technique.

*Permanent address: Pharmacological Research Centre, Chemical Works of GEDEON Richter Ltd., P.O. Box 27, Budapest 10, H-1475 Hungary.

Materials and Methods

All procedures were approved by the Committee of Animal Bio-Ethics of the University of Groningen. Five male Wistar rats (locally bred at the Central Animal Facility, Groningen) were housed individually and fed ad libitum in a temperature- and light-controlled room (Light/Dark: 7.00/19.00 h). Two microdialysis probes were stereotaxically implanted in the bilateral hippocampus under pentobarbital anaesthesia, as described [13]. Twenty-four to 48 h later the first microdialysis experiments were performed, and glucose containing or lacking perfusion fluids were perfused for 2.5 h at random order. During perfusion the rats were stressed by immobilization for 10 min by keeping them upside down in the hand [13]. Every 5 min a dialysate was collected from the rat (flow 3 µL/min obtained by a pump; CMA 100, Carnegie Medicine, Stockholm, Sweden). At the end of the measurement the samples were stored at −25°C until analysis. The rats were housed for another 12 or 13 days, and similar perfusion experiments were performed (with or without glucose-containing media and immobilization stress). All 5 animals underwent the same perfusion and stress procedures. The next day the rats were killed for histology. Prior to transcardial perfusion rats were deeply anaesthetized with pentobarbital (50 mg/kg i.p.) and perfused with 0.9% saline for one minute, followed by 4% paraformaldehyde in 0.1 M phosphate buffer (pH 7.4) for 10 min. Brains were processed as described [14, 25]. Lactate was electrochemically detected on-line after enzymic oxidation as described [18]. Biochemical data are presented $\mu M \pm SEM$. To compare data the Student-t-test was used. Significance was taken at $p < 0.05$. Representative examples of the histological observations are shown.

Results

An example of a recording of dialysate samples collected before and during stress is shown in Fig. 1. Extracellular hippocampus lactate tended to be higher in the absence of 5 µM glucose in the acute preparation, whereas in the chronic preparation lactate was 10–20 fold higher in the presence of glucose (Fig. 2). The stress effects were significant in the acute preparation both

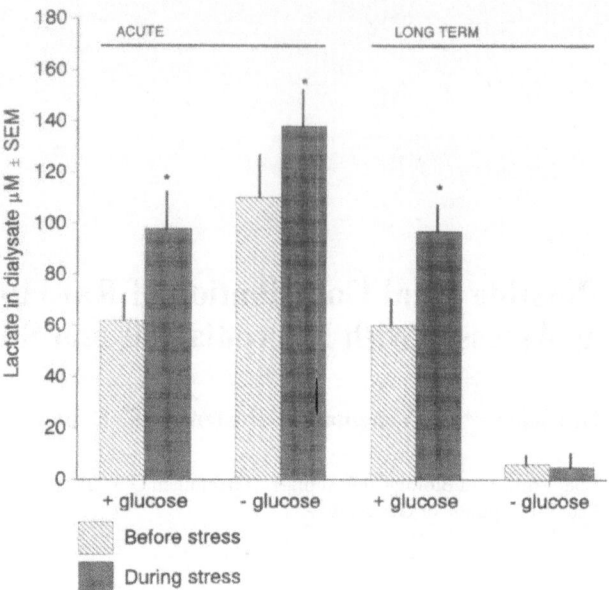

Fig. 2. Baseline 10–15 min before stress and taken 10–15 min after the onset of stress. Stress affected levels of hippocampus extracellular lactate of rats with dialysis probes implanted 1 or 2 days (acute) or 13/14 days (long term) earlier. Data of 5 rats; * indicates significant increases (p < 0.05) from baseline levels. In the absence of glucose, the baseline levels of lactate were significantly higher in the acute experiments whereas these levels were significantly lower in the chronic experiments (p < 0.05)

in the presence and the absence of glucose, whereas in the long-term preparation the increase in lactate during stress was significant only in the presence of glucose.

Figure 3 shows GFAP staining at several magnifications. Near the probe there is a clear increase in the density of GFAP positive cells (Fig. 3A, B, D), as compared to stained control tissue (Fig. 3C). In the chronic preparation there is damage in the bilateral corpus callosum (Fig. 4A), the hippocampus and cerebral cortex adjacent to the probe. Such damage was neither present in the acute preparations nor in control tissue (Fig. 4C).

Discussion

Both in the present study and that of Fellows *et al.* [7] omission of glucose resulted in an increase in the concentration of extracellular lactate in the acute preparation. Fellows *et al.* [7] suggest that high glucose concentration results in a block of K_{ATP} channels, thus leading to decreased lactate levels, as was supported by their results with tolbutamide, as well. Massive lactate efflux obtained with astrocyte cultures in the absence of glucose [3, 4] has been explained by the breakdown of glycogen. Previously [12], a paradigm similar to

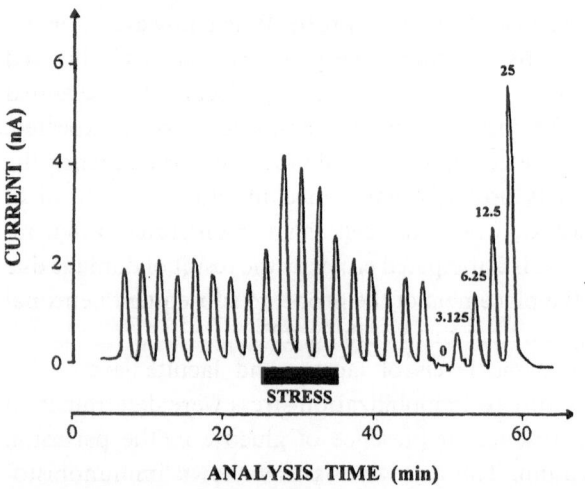

Fig. 1. The lactate of the stressed rat was recorded 2 days after implantation of the probe in the absence of glucose in the perfusate. The bar indicates the duration of the immobilization stress (10 min)

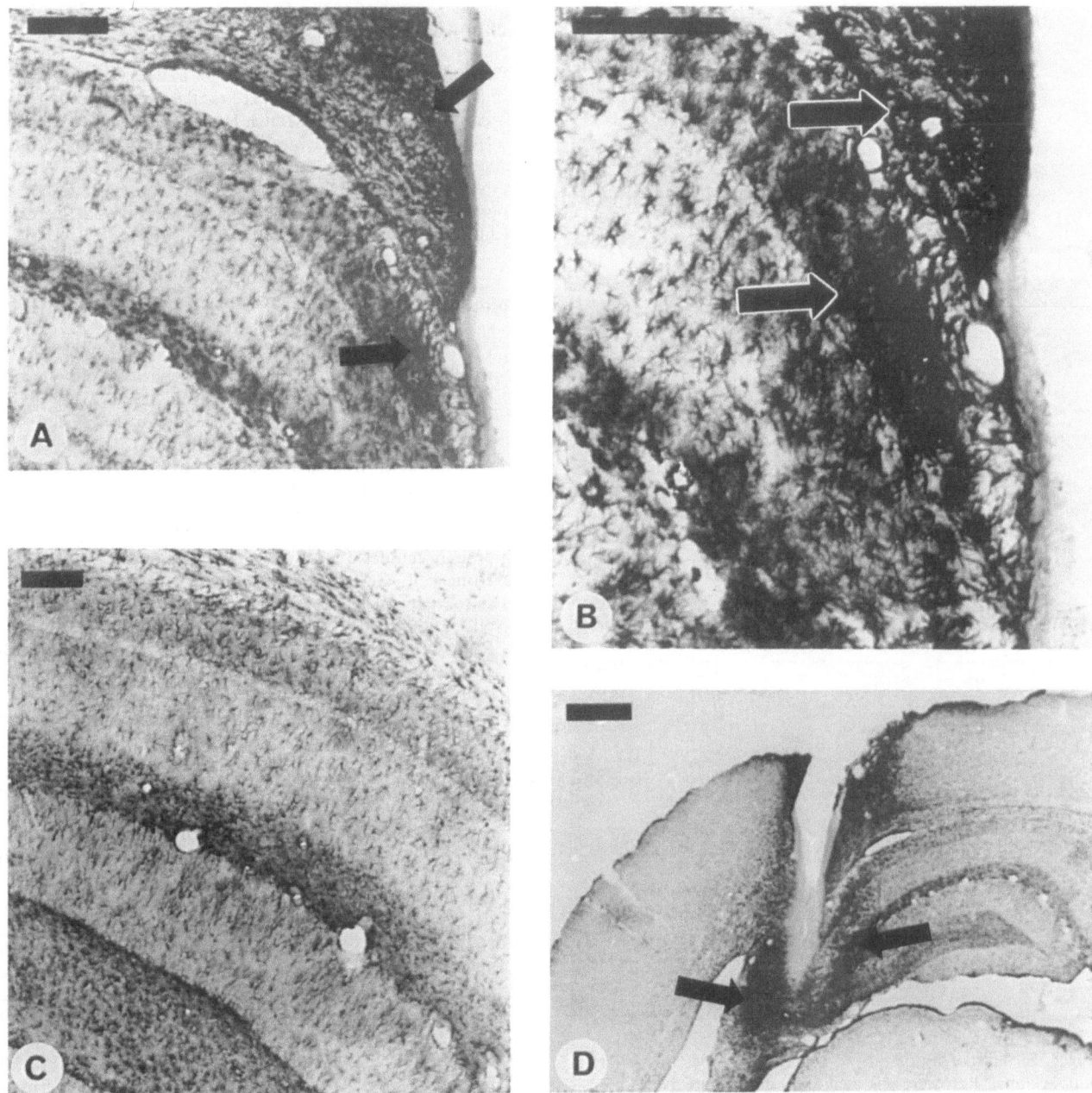

Fig. 3. Immunocytochemical staining for GFAP of the hippocampus sections obtained from rats 14 days after placement of the dialysis probe. Density around the probe (A, B and D) is far higher than in control tissue (C) or farther removed from the probe (B,D). The bar corresponds to 200 µm in A, B and C; and 0.5 mm in D. The location of the probe is indicated with arrows

that of the present study was used to distinguish the cellular compartments of potassium-induced release of neurotransmitters and related compounds in micro-dialysates. In the acute but not in the chronic preparation the release of neurotransmitters, such as GABA, glutamate and aspartate was high when exposed to potassium at high concentrations, whereas the response of taurine did not differ in either preparations. These results emphasize the importance of potassium

channels in non-neuronal cells in the cellular efflux of endogenous metabolites including taurine. Therefore, non-neuronal activity of K_{ATP} channels may contribute to the effects of tolbutamide reported by Fellows et al. [7]. During the present long-term preparation the glucose dependency is reversed: there is not only a large increase in baseline levels of lactate in the presence of glucose, but also the stress effects were restored. These results are consistent with the idea that there is insuffi-

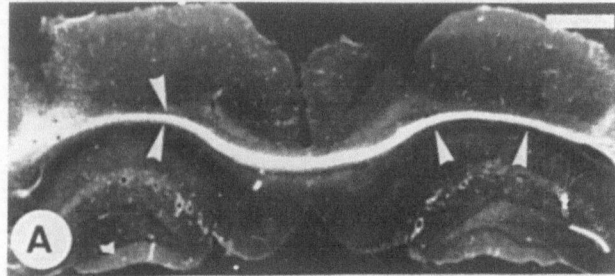

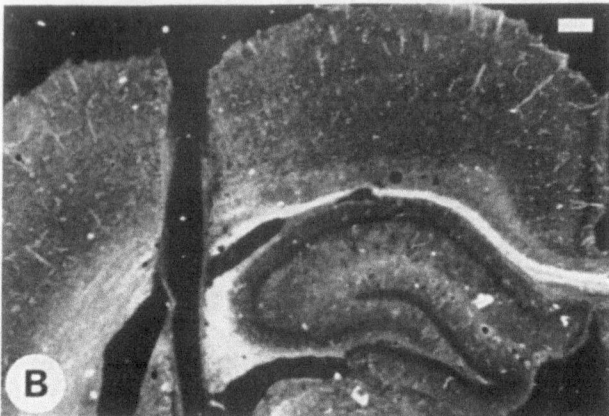

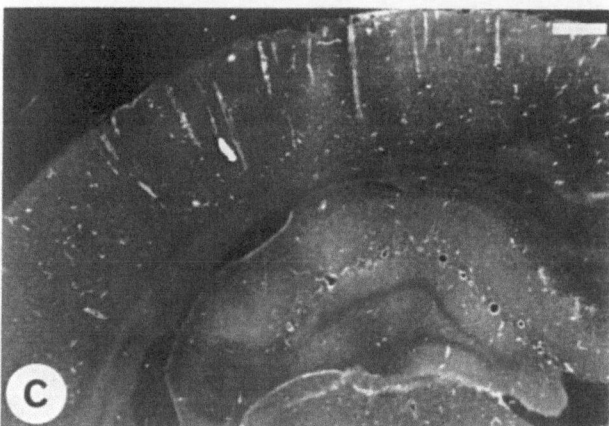

Fig. 4. Silver staining of rats with bilateral probes in the lateral hippocampus. Rats were operated on 14 days before fixation. Positive staining was seen in the corpus callosum (A), the cerebral cortex and near the probe (B), but was absent in control tissue (C). The bars indicate 0.4 mm. Arrows indicate silver-stained degenerative processes

cient glucose in the circulation to reach the tissue around the dialysis probe so glycogen stores are depleted.

Interestingly, in the presence of glucose the tissue is reactive to mild stress, indicating that the tissue around the probe is viable. So, if the conclusion of the present study is that a substantial proportion of extracellular lactate (if not all) is derived from non-neuronal compartments, in particular glial cells, stress activates such compartments via neurotransmitter related processes.

Acknowledgements

The authors thank Ms. M.G. Bixel for evaluation of the manuscript. Ms. Joke Venema typed and edited the text. Financial support has been obtained from the Dutch Heart Foundation (Zoetemeer, the Netherlands), the Saal van Zwanenburg Foundation (Oss, the Netherlands), the Dutch Technology Foundation (STW, Utrecht, the Netherlands), the Nuffic organisation for a student exchange programme (The Hague, The Netherlands) and the J.K. de Cock Stichting (Groningen, The Netherlands).

References

1. DeBruin LA, Schasfoort EMC, Steffens AB, Korf J (1990) Extracellular lactate during stress and exercise measured in the rat hippocampus and striatum. Am J Physiol 259: R773–R779
2. Dijk S, Krugers HJ, Korf J (1991) The effect of theophylline and immobilization stress on haloperidol-induced catalepsy and on metabolism in striatum and hippocampus, studied with lactography. Neuropharmacology 30: 469–473
3. Dringen R, Hamprecht B (1993) Inhibition by 2-deoxyglucose and 1,5-gluconolactone of glycogen mobilization in astroglia-rich primary cultures. J Neurochem 60: 1498–1504
4. Dringen R, Gebhardt R, Hamprecht B (1993) Glycogen in astrocytes: possible function as lactate supply for neighbouring cells. Brain Res 623: 208–214
5. Fellows LK, Boutelle MG, Fillenz M (1992) Extracellular brain glucose levels reflect local neuronal activity: a microdialysis study in awake, freely moving rats. J Neurochem 59: 2141–2147
6. Fellows LK, Boutelle MG, Fillenz M (1993a) Physiological stimulation increases nonoxidative glucose metabolism in the brain of the freely moving rat. J Neurochem 60: 1258–1263
7. Fellows LK, Boutelle MG, Fillenz M (1993b) ATP-sensitive potassium channels and local energy demands in the rat hippocampus: an in vivo study. J Neurochem 61: 949–954
8. Georgieva J, Luthman J, Mohringe B, Magnusson O (1993) Tissue and microdialysate changes after repeated and permanent probe implantation in the striatum of freely moving rats. Brain Res Bull 31: 463–470
9. Hallstrom A, Carlsson A, Hillered L, Ungerstedt U (1989) Simultaneous determination of lactate, pyruvate and ascorbate in microdialysis samples from rat brain, blood, fat, and muscle using high performance liquid chromatography. J Pharmacol Meth 22: 113–123
10. Katayama Y, Kawamata T, Kano T, Tsubokawa T (1992) Excitatory amino acid antagonist administered via microdialysis attenuates lactate accumulation during cerebral ischemia and subsequent hippocampal damage. Brain Res 586: 329–333
11. Korf J, DeBoer J (1990) Lactography as an approach to monitor glucose metabolism on-line in brain and muscle. Int J Biochem 22: 1371–1379
12. Korf J, Venema K (1985) Amino acids in rat striatal dialysates: methodological aspects and changes after electroconvulsive shock. J Neurochem 45: 1341–1348
13. Krugers HJ, Jaarsma D, Korf J (1992) Rat hippocampal lactate efflux during electroconvulsive shock is differently dependent on entorhinal cortex and adrenal integrity. J Neurochem 58: 826–830
14. Krugers HJ, Medema RM, Postema F, Korf J (1994) Induction of glial fibrillary acidic protein (GFAP)-immunoreactivity in the rat dentate gyrus after adrenalectomy: Comparison with neurodegenerative changes using silver impregnation. Hippocampus 4: 307–314
15. Kuhr WG, Korf J (1988) Extracellular lactic acid as an indicator of brain metabolism: continuous on-line measurement in con-

scious, freely moving rats with intrastriatal dialysis. J Cereb Blood Flow Metab 8: 130–137

16. Kuhr WG, VandenBerg CJ, Korf J (1988) In vivo identification and quantitative evaluation of carrier mediated transport of lactate at the cellular level in the striatum of conscious, freely moving rats. J Cereb Blood Flow Metab 9: 848–856

17. Kurosawa M, Hallstrom A, Ungerstedt U (1991) Changes in cerebral blood flow do not directly affect in vivo recovery of extracellular lactate through microdialysis. Neurosci Lett 126: 123–126

18. Middelveld R, De Groote C, DeBoer J, Venema K, Korf J (1994) Monitoring of lactate using microdialysis: animal studies and clinical applications. Biol Ital 24: 21–25

19. Pellerin L, Magistretti PJ (1994) glutamate uptake into astrocytes stimulates aerobic glycolysis: a mechanism coupling neuronal activity to glucose utilization. Proc Natl Acad Sci USA 91(22): 10625–10629

20. Pfeiffer B, Elmer K, Roggendorf W, Hamprecht B, (1990) Immunohistochemical demonstration of glycogen phosphorylase in rat brain slices. Histochemistry 94: 73–80

21. Schasfoort EMC, DeBruin LA, Korf J (1988) Mild stress stimulates rat hippocampal glucose utilization transiently via NMDA receptors, as assessed by lactography. Brain Res 475: 58–63

22. Schurr A, West CA, Rigor BM (1988) Lactate-supported synaptic function in the rat hippocampal slice preparation. Science 250: 1326–1328

23. Shuaib A, Xu K, Siren A-L, Feuerstein G, Hallenbeck J, Davis JN (1990) Assessment of damage from implantation of microdialysis probes in the rat hippocampus with silver impregnation staining. Neurosci Lett 112: 149–154

24. Takita M, Mikuni M, Takahashi K (1992) Habituation of lactate release to stress stimuli in rat prefrontal cortex in vivo. Am J Physiol 263: R722–R727

25. Ter Horst GJ, Knollema S, Knigge MF, Kruger HJ, Postema F, Hom HW (1995) Selective silver staining for demonstrating degenerating neurons. In: Wouterlood FG (ed) Neuroscience protocols, Vol 50. Elsevier, Amsterdam, pp 1–13

26. Tildon JT, McKenna MC, Stevenson J, Couto R (1993) Transport of L-lactate by cultured rat brain astrocytes. Neurochem Res 18: 177–184

Correspondence: J. Korf, M.D., Department of Biological psychiatry, Groningen University, P.O. Box 30.001, NL 9700 RB Groningen, The Netherlands.

Acta Neurochir (1996) [Suppl] 67: 6–12
© Springer-Verlag 1996

Application of Glutamate in the Cortex of Rats: A Microdialysis Study

B. Alessandri[1], **H. Landolt**[3], **H. Langemann**[1], **J. Gregorin**, **J. Hall**, and **O. Gratzl**[2]

[1]Neurosurgery Laboratory, Department of Research, [2]Neurosurgery Clinic, Cantonal Hospital Basel, Basel, and [3]Cantonal Hospital Aarau, Neurosurgery Department, Aarau, Switzerland

Summary

Glutamate, a major neurotransmitter in the brain, is also involved in pathophysiological processes resulting in secondary lesions following ischaemia or trauma. In the present study we investigated the relationship between glutamate excitotoxicity, free radical induction (indicated by ascorbic acid level) and glucose-lactate metabolism. Monosodium glutamate was applied through microdialysis probes (500 mM in perfusate) into the cortex of rats for 30 minutes and ascorbic acid (ASC), glucose (GLUC) and lactate (LAC) were measured in dialysates. Glutamate produced a cortical lesion with an average volume of $12.7 \pm 1.4 \, mm^3$. Analysis of dialysates revealed a significant increase of ASC ($325 \pm 52\%$ of baseline) and LAC ($677 \pm 86\%$) in the core lesion. In the lesion periphery a nonsignificant and short-lasting elevation was measured for both parameters with a second microdialysis probe (about 1.3 mm frontally to the first probe). A concomitant decrease of GLUC was found in both probes, reaching $29 \pm 8\%$ and $60 \pm 7\%$ of basal levels in the core and periphery of the lesion, respectively. In addition, we studied the delivery characteristics of several glutamate concentrations (10, 100 or 1000 mM in perfusate) during a 90-minute application into the cortex. The delivery of glutamate from the perfusate to the brain was about 33–38% in the first 30 min and afterwards 11–25% of the total in the perfusate. The results show that cortical application of glutamate changes the composition of the extracellular fluid, which could contribute to the development of the lesion.

Keywords: Glutamate excitotoxicity; ascorbic acid; glucose metabolism; microdialysis.

Introduction

Although there have recently been great improvements in the treatment of patients in the neurosurgical critical care unit, there are still many cases of delayed secondary damage to the injured brain, leading to a worsened outcome or even death. Postmortem investigation in such cases shows the presence of lesions in the cortex which have been called "ischaemic" [12]. However, the real cause of these lesions has not yet been elucidated. They are known to occur even when cerebral perfusion pressure (CPP) is adequate, so that classic ischaemia cannot be the sole cause.

It is known that the neurotransmitter aminoacid glutamate is excitotoxic both in vitro in neuronal cell cultures [6] and in vivo (e.g. [26]). Microdialytic studies in animal models have shown that levels of glutamate increase markedly in the extracellular fluid (ECF) after trauma (e.g. [28]), acute subdural haematoma [5] and focal ischaemia (e.g. [7]). These increases result in excessive activation of glutamate receptors, which might initiate a cascade of neurochemical events leading to cell death. It is therefore of interest that glutamate receptor antagonists have shown efficacy in the treatment of ischaemic lesions (e.g. [2]).

However, there is still a discussion about the role played by glutamate in the pathogenesis of delayed lesions. In addition, there is not much known about neurochemical processes which are directly initiated by glutamate in vivo. Therefore we used an in vivo model of glutamate neurotoxicity in which glutamate was applied to the cortex of rats through a microdialysis probe, producing a dose-dependent lesion [3, 10, 20]. Glutamate itself was chosen instead of another excitotoxic amino acid such as kainic acid or N-methyl-D-aspartate because glutamate is the endogenous neurotransmitter in the brain. It activates all glutamate receptor subtypes and is the natural substrate for the high affinity uptake mechanism of neurons and glial cells. In addition, a recent study showed that the cerebral blood flow does not fall below the noxious level following glutamate application [10]. Therefore the effects of excessive extracellular glutamate can be distinguished from those of ischaemia. In this study we have used this model to examine the effects of increased ECF glutamate on energy status (glucose, lactate) and on the antioxidant ascorbic acid in the cortex; in addition, results of histological investigations of the glutamate lesion and experiments to estimate the amount of glutamate delivered to the brain are reported.

Methods and Material

Microdialysis

The experiments were carried out with 17 male Sprague-Dawley rats (weight ca. 280 g). Anaesthesia was induced by flooding the cage with 3% Halothane in oxygen for several minutes. The animal was then fixed in a stereotactic frame and general anaesthesia was continued with 0.8 to 1.5% Halothane in oxygen. An arterial line was established (canulation of the femoral artery) to monitor mean arterial blood pressure (MABP) and to collect blood samples which were analyzed for blood gases, pH and plasma glucose.

All apparatus required for the microdialysis was purchased from CMA/M Microdialysis (Stockholm, Sweden). The microdialysis system was perfused with Ringer solution (NaCl 155 mM, KCl 4 mM, NaHCO$_3$ 1 mM, CaCl$_2$ 2.75 mM, pH 7.1) at a flow rate of 2 µl/min and dialysates were collected at 15 or 30 min intervals. The probe for application of glutamate (probe A; CMLA/12, 3 or 4mm membrane) was implanted into the left frontoparietal cortex (AP = 0–1 mm, ML = 4 mm to bregma, DV = 5mm; angle = 17°), and a second similar probe for monitoring (probe M) was implanted at a distance of 1.2–1.4 mm frontally from the first one. Both probes were initially perfused for 2–3 hours to allow equilibration. Then probe A was perfused for 30 min with Ringer solution containing monosodium glutamate (500 mM). Microdialysis samples were collected from both probes for a further 3 hrs. The animals were decapitated before they regained consciousness. The brains were immediately removed, frozen to −20° in isopentane and stored at −80°C.

Histology

Haemotoxylin-eosin staining: Sections of 10 µm were prepared in a cryostat. They were taken every 100–200 µm throughout the lesion (visually controlled) and stained with hematoxylin (Meyer's hemalum solution, E. Merck, Switzerland) and eosin (Fluka, Switzerland). Morphometric determination of the lesion volume was performed with an electronic image analysis system. The study was approved by the Cantonal Ethics Committee of Basel.

Analysis of Dialysates and Blood Samples

Dialysates were analysed for ASC, GLUC and LAC. GLUC and LAC were analysed as previously described [21, 22]. Briefly, GLUC was quantified in dialysates (15–20 µl) and blood samples (5–10 µl) by a colorimetric enzymatic method using a kit (Trinder from Sigma). LAC was also determined enzymatically using lactate dehydrogenase (fluorometrical measurement of NAD$^+$) in 15–20 µl of the dialysate. The antioxidant ASC was measured in 10–20 µl of dialysates by HPLC as described previously [17, 23]. All values are given as mean ± s.e.m. Basal level was calculated as the mean of the last two (ASC) or three samples (GLUC, LAC) before glutamate application.

Glutamate Delivery Characteristics

In a separate study the diffusion characteristics of three concentrations of monosodium glutamate in the cortex of rats were investigated [20]. A microdialysis probe (CMA/12, 4 mm membrane) was inserted into the rat brain as described above. After equilibration the probe was perfused for 90 min with mock cerebrospinal fluid (CSF; NaCl 135 mM, KCl 1 mM, KH$_2$PO$_4$ 2 mM, CaCl$_2$ 1.2 mM, MgCl$_2$ 1 mM, pH 7.4) containing 10, 100 or 1000 mM monosodium glutamate at a flow rate of 2 µl/min. The amount of glutamate delivered to the tissue was estimated from the ratio of outlet and inlet concentrations. Glutamate in the collected fractions was analysed by HPLC using a gradient elution profile. It was detected as its fluorescent derivative (excitation wavelength 230 nm, emission wavelength > 400 nm) following pre-column derivatization with orthophthaldialdehyde.

Statistics

Statistical analysis was performed using the data analysis package StatView 4.02 (Abacus Concepts Inc., USA, 1993). Baseline value and values after glutamate treatment were compared using an analysis of variance followed by posthoc Bonferroni/Dunnet t-tests. Significance level was $p < 0.05$. Values are given as mean ± s.e.m.

Results

Physiological Parameters

Blood gases (pO$_2$, pCO$_2$), blood pH and mean arterial blood pressure were within physiological ranges. Average blood glucose was also not affected by glutamate application (Fig. 3).

Histology

A typical lesion produced by 500 mM monosodium glutamate in the perfusate (applied for 30 min) and the average morphometrically assessed lesion volume are shown in Fig. 1. Around the probe, a pale lesion with

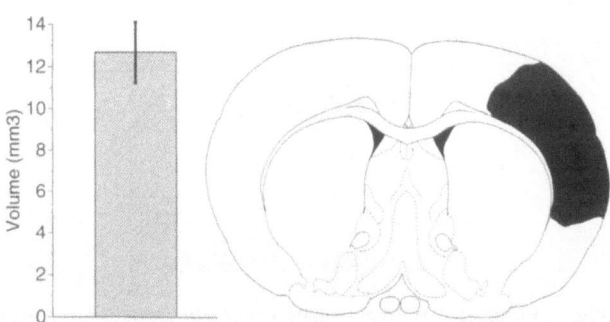

Fig. 1. Mean lesion volume (left, n = 7) and schematic drawing (right) of a coronal section with the maximal lesion area (rat #6) produced by 500 mM glutamate in the perfusate. Glutamate was applied through microdialysis probes into the cortex of rats during 30 minutes. The animals were decapitated 3 hours after the start of glutamate application

a marked boundary was produced in the cortex. The lesion extended anteriorly and posteriorly (1.93 ± 0.12 mm in each direction) and had a volume of 12.67 ± 1.43 mm³ (n = 7). The histopathological features in the area of pallor have previously been described [20], i.e. triangulation of the nucleus, shrinkage of neurons and neurophil, and swelling of perineuronal astrocytes. Histological examination also showed that in most cases the M-probe was positioned inside the boundary of the lesion.

Ascorbic Acid

Dialysates of 10 animals were analysed for ASC. Dialysates from the M-probe of two animals were lost because of technical problems. The time-courses of ASC in the dialysates from the application (A-) and the monitoring (M-) probes are shown in Fig. 2. In the last dialysate sample of baseline equilibration ASC levels of the A- and M-probe were 5.33 ± 2.2 μM (101 ± 6% of basal level) and 4.44 ± 1.3 μM, (84 ± 8% of basal level), respectively. Fifteen minutes after the start of glutamate application, the levels of ASC in the dialysate of the A-probe started to increase, reaching a peak after 60 minutes (10.7 ± 2 μM). ASC was significantly increased in the dialysates of the A-probe compared to the baseline until the end of the experiment. In the dialysates of the M-probe, ASC started to increase

slightly after 45 min, reaching the highest level of 5.63 μM after 75 min (not significant compared to baseline).

Glucose and Lactate

The effects of glutamate on GLUC and LAC levels in the dialysates were investigated in 7 animals (Fig. 3). From levels of about 352 ± 33 μM (last sample before glutamate; 95 ± 6% of basal level) and 344 ± 20 μM (100 ± 4%) in dialysates from the A- and M-probes, respectively, GLUC markedly decreased following the start of glutamate application. The lowest GLUC levels were 113 ± 34 μM (29 ± 8%) at 90 minutes (A-

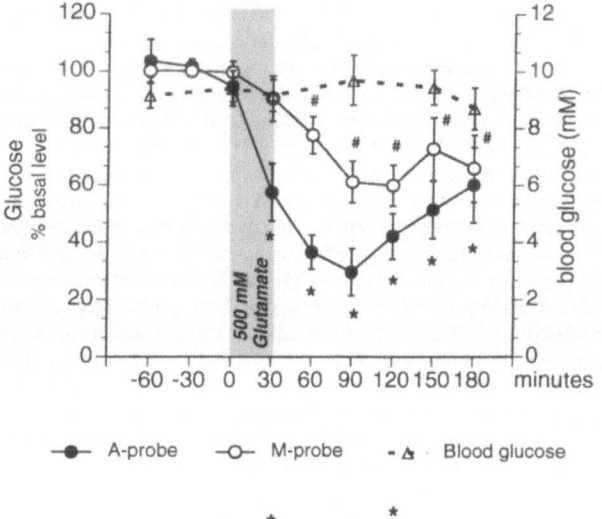

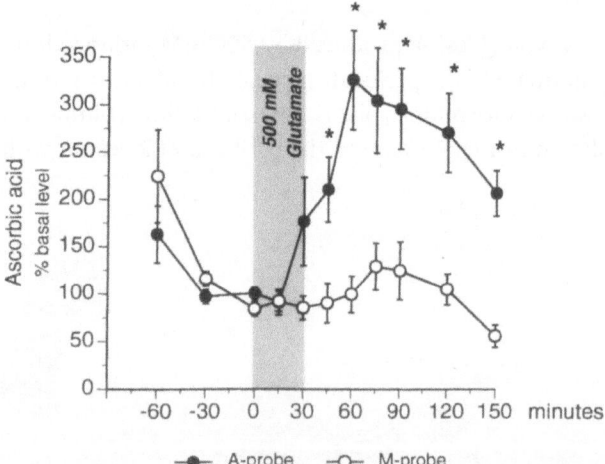

Fig. 2. Effects of 500 mM glutamate in the perfusate on ascorbic acid (ASC) in cortical dialysates of rats. Glutamate was delivered through an application probe (A-probe). A monitoring probe (M-probe) was placed at a distance of about 1.3 mm from the A-probe. Mean basal level (average of last two values before glutamate) was compared with each time-point during and after glutamate application using an analysis of variance with posthoc Bonferroni/Dunnet t-test comparisons (*p < 0.05)

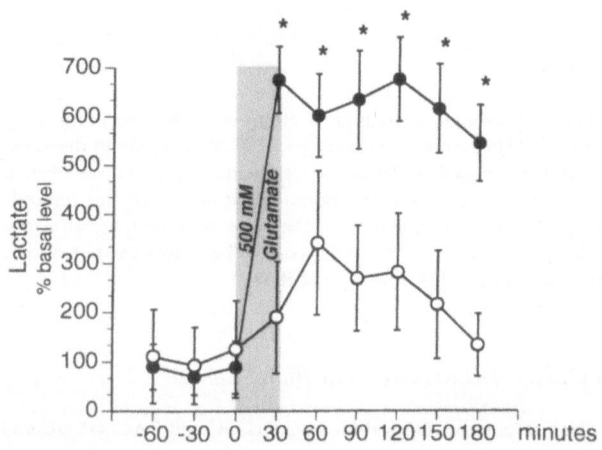

Fig. 3. Effects of 500 mM glutamate in the perfusate on glucose (GLUC, upper graph) and lactate (LAC, lower graph) in cortical dialysates of rats. Glutamate was delivered through an application probe (A-probe). A monitoring probe (M-probe) was placed at a distance of about 1.3 mm from the A-probe. Mean basal level (average of last three values before glutamate) was compared with each time-point during and after glutamate application using an analysis of variance with posthoc Bonferroni/Dunnet t-test comparisons (*,#p < 0.05)

probe) and $191 \pm 16\,\mu M$ ($60 \pm 7\%$) at 120 minutes (M-probe). At the end of the experiment, GLUC levels in both probes were about 60% of basal level, but still significantly different from baseline. Already in the first sample following the start of glutamate application, there was a massive increase in LAC from a level of $64 \pm 38\,\mu M$ to $486 \pm 62\,\mu M$ in the A-probe (Fig. 4b). LAC stayed at this high level throughout the experiment. There were significant differences to baseline values at all time-points. LAC was slightly but not significantly increased in the dialysates from the M-probe ($75 \pm 59\,\mu M$ before and $205 \pm 88\,\mu M$ after glutamate).

Glutamate Delivery Characteristic

The diffusion rate for glutamate is shown in Fig. 4. Mean percentage ($\pm$ s.d.) of total glutamate delivered to the brain was about 35% during the first 30 minutes for 10, 100, and 1000 mM and decreased to $11\% \pm 10$, $18\% \pm 14$, and $19\% \pm 6$, respectively, during the second 30 minutes of sampling. At 1000 mM the amount of glutamate delivered from the perfusate to the brain continued to decrease during the last 30 minutes of glutamate perfusion ($11\% \pm 3$), whereas a slight increase was observed at the two lower concentrations (16 ± 14, $25\% \pm 14$).

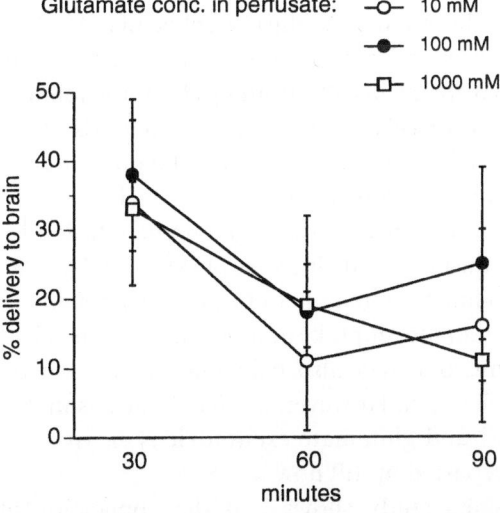

Fig. 4. In vivo delivery characteristics of 10, 100, or 1000mM glutamate in the perfusate. Glutamate was applied through microdialysis probes into the cortex of rats for 90 minutes. Delivery was calculated from the difference between glutamate concentrations in perfusates and collected dialysates. Values are given as mean $\pm$ s.d. (5 rats/concentration)

Discussion

The present data show that the cortical application of glutamate produces large lesions, induces the release of ASC and leads to a decrease of GLUC and to an increase of LAC in cortical dialysates.

Glutamate Lesion and Delivery

The application of glutamate through microdialysis probes was reported by several authors. In these studies, however, glutamate was applied for 90 minutes to the cortex [4, 10, 20] or for 120 minutes to the striatum [3, 19]. The cortical administration of 10–1000 mM monosodium glutamate for 90 minutes led to dose-dependent lesions which were histologically similar to those seen after ischaemia, with a threshold concentration between 10 and 100 mM glutamate in the perfusate [4, 20]. In the present study it could be shown that glutamate application for only 30 minutes, mimicking the time-course of glutamate release during ischaemia (e.g. [35]), already results in large lesions. From the 500 mM glutamate in the perfusate, about 35% actually diffused into the cortex during 30 minutes, which would give a maximal extracellular concentration of about 200 mM. However, such high concentrations would not be reached in the perifocal region of the lesion. Assuming a threshold concentration between 10 and 100 mM glutamate in the perfusate and a 35% delivery of glutamate to the brain, it can be suggested that the necessary extracellular levels have to reach about 4 to 40 mM in order to produce lesions. Calculated extracellular peak levels of glutamate following ischaemia may reach 4 mM [2], or even higher. Recently, we could show that under certain conditions (e.g. disturbed ion homeostasis) a non-lesion producing glutamate concentration of 10 mM in the perfusate can produce lesions [1].

Effects on Ascorbate, Glucose and Lactate

From animal models of ischaemia it is known that occlusion of the middle cerebral artery (MCAO) leads to an elevation of ASC [15] and LAC [14] and to a decrease of GLUC levels [24] in dialysates. Similar effects were also found during brain retraction in aneurysm operations (see Mendelowitsch *et al.*, this volume). In one head-injured patient, we also found changes of ASC levels over time [22]. Thus, these parameters could possibly be used as indicators of secondary brain tissue damage. Since glutamate release after brain injury or ischaemia may also contribute to the production of secondary lesions, changes in extracellular levels of ASC, GLUC and LAC were investigated after glutamate application into the cortex of rats.

Ascorbic acid has been shown to play an important role in the defense reaction against free radicals [18], which are increased under ischaemic conditions [11]. Although there is a decrease of whole brain tissue content of ASC after MCAO [25], a local extracellular increase was found in the core of ischaemic lesions [15]. This is of special interest because ASC may also initiate lipid peroxidation (see [13]) and was found to be neurotoxic in vitro. It was recently found that intrastriatal injections of kainic acid or N-methyl-D-aspartate resulted in ASC release [36] similar to that found after glutamate. ASC is released from glutamatergic neurons as part of the glutamate reuptake process, in which the high-affinity glutamate transporter exchanges ASC for glutamate (see [13] for a recent review). In addition to glutamate-induced ascorbate release, ASC might leak from intracellular compartments after perforation of membranes by lipid peroxidation and following cell death. This would be in accordance with the activation of free radical production (measured as 2,5-dihydroxybenzoic acid) by intrastriatal glutamate application [3, 19]. Whether free radicals are able to stimulate ASC release directly is not known. However, the pathophysiological consequences of elevated extracellular ASC during glutamate application or ischaemia are not clear at the moment and more experiments will be necessary to clarify its role in glutamate excitotoxicity.

Glucose is the major energy substrate for the brain. In a recent animal study it has been shown that GLUC is also important for the reuptake of glutamate, which is released during ischemia. A low extracellular GLUC level leads to an about 7-fold higher glutamate level in dialyates than a high GLUC level [34]. This is supported by in vitro findings demonstrating that glutamate becomes neurotoxic to cerebellar neurons when intracellular GLUC levels are reduced [29]. These results are important since permanent ischaemia results in a massive reduction in extracellular GLUC [24] which would facilitate extracellular accumulation of neurotoxic amounts of glutamate.

The present data show that the application of glutamate through a microdialysis probe reduced extracellular GLUC content in the core and, to a lesser extent, also towards its periphery. In previous studies GLUC utilization and cerebral blood flow were measured with

2-deoxyglucose [4] and with ^{14}C- iodoantipyrine (see [10]), respectively, after glutamate application. Glutamate decreased GLUC utilization in the centre of the lesion and increased it in the boundary zone. At the same time, cerebral blood flow was maintained above 50 mg/min/100g brain tissue, which is not considered to be harmful for brain functions. Several mechanisms seem to be involved in the immediate decrease of local extracellular GLUC levels, namely the massive neuronal activation (e.g. [8]), the reuptake of glutamate into glial cell and neurons [27, 34], and the reduced blood flow within the lesion (e.g. [31]). Contrary to a persistent GLUC decrease during permanent MCAO [24], the local application of glutamate only led to a temporary extracellular GLUC reduction. This might be best explained by a reduced GLUC need because of developing tissue damage, and a maintained blood flow with GLUC delivery even to the core of the lesion.

Lactate: Another important finding in our study is the immediate increase of LAC in dialysates concomitant with the GLUC decrease. In a recent paper, it was suggested that nonoxidative metabolism of GLUC may be required to meet high-energy needs quickly, such as fuelling the NA^+/K^+-ATPase to restore ionic gradients during neuronal activation (e.g glutamate stimulation of neurons; reuptake of glutamate into glial cells and neurons) [9]. LAC produced within the brain can be used from cells as energy substrate and might become an important energy substrate in ischaemia [30]. On the other hand, high levels of LAC, which have been recorded during ischaemia [14] lead to lactacidosis and are involved in the formation of intracellular edema in cell cultures [33], mitochondrial damage [16] or cell death (see [32]). Acidosis of the extracellular fluid also provides a very favourable environment for free radical formation, which has been shown to occur during striatal glutamate infusion [3, 19]. Thus, the immediate increase of extracellular LAC following glutamate may help to provide enough energy for glutamate reuptake or other energy-dependent mechanisms, but may also contribute to glutamate-induced cell death. However, a direct relationship between LAC and glutamate excitotoxicity in vivo has not been reported up till now.

The present study shows that the application of glutamate produces changes in metabolism of glucose and free radical scavengers, reflected as an alteration in the composition of the extracellular fluid. Thus, glutamate application leads to histological and neurochemical findings similar in some respects to those seen during focal ischaemia, without any noxious reduction of cerebral blood flow. Since the extracellular concentration of glutamate during ischaemia or trauma is much lower than the concentration achieved in this study, further investigation will be necessary to show whether the reported changes in the extracellular fluid composition or other factors such as spreading depression or ion shifts could potentiate or inhibit glutamate excitotoxicity in this model.

Acknowledgement

This study was supported by the Swiss National Science Foundation (grant #31-36476.92) and the Swiss Academy of Medical Sciences.

References

1. Alessandri B, Landolt H, Langemann H, Gratzl O (1995) Peracute effects of microdialytically applied glutamate in the cortex of rats. J Cereb Blood Flow Metab 15: S420
2. Benveniste H (1991) The excitotoxin hypothesis in relation to cerebral ischemia. Cerebrovasc Brain Metab Rev 3: 213–245
3. Boisvert DPJ, Schreiber C (1992) Interrelationship of excitotoxic and free radical mechanisms In: Krieglstein J, Oberpichler-Schwenk H (eds) 4th Symposium on Pharmacology of Cerebral Ischemia. Medpharm, Stuttgart, pp 311–320
4. Bullock R, Landolt H, Fujisawa H (1993) Pattern of increased glucose use after extracellular glutamate infusion. J Cereb Blood Flow Metab 13 [Suppl 1]: S578
5. Chen MH, Bullock R, Graham DI, Miller JD, McCulloch J (1991) Ischemic neuronal damage after acute subdural hematoma in the rat—effects of pretreatment with a glutamate antagonist. J Neurosurg 74: 944–950
6. Choi DW, Maulucci-Gedde MA, Kriegstein AR (1987) Glutamate neurotoxicity in cortical cell culture. J Neurosci 7: 357–368
7. Drejer J, Benveniste H, Diemer NH, Schousboe A (1985) Cellular origin of ischemia-induced glutamate release from brain tissue in vivo and in vitro. J Neurochem 45: 145–151
8. Fellows LK, Boutelle MG, Fillenz M (1992) Extracellular brain glucose levels reflect local neuronal activity: a microdialysis study in awake, freely moving rats. J Neurochem 59: 2141–2147
9. Fellows LK, Boutelle MG, Fillenz M (1993) Physiological stimulation increases nonoxidative glucose metabolism in the brain of freely moving rats. J Neurochem 60: 1258
10. Fujisawa H, Dawson D, Browne SE, MacKay KB, Bullock R, McCulloch J (1993) Pharmacological modification of glutamate neurotoxicity in vivo. Brain Res 629: 73–78
11. Ginsberg MD, Globus MY-T, Martinez e, Morimoto T, Lin B, Schnippering H, Alonso OF, Busto R (1994) Oxygen radical and excitotoxic processes in brain ischemia and trauma. In: Krieglstein J, Oberpichler–Schwenk H (eds) 4th Symposium on Pharmacology of Cerebral Ischemia. Medpharm, Stuttgart, Marburg, Germany, pp 255–268
12. Graham DI, Ford I, Adams JH, Doyle D, Teasdale GM, Lawrence AE, McLellan DR (1989) Ischaemic brain damage is still common in fatal non-missile head injury. J Neurol Neurosurg Psychiatry 52: 346–350
13. Grünewald RA (1993) Ascorbic acid in the brain. Brain Res Rev 18: 123–133
14. Hillered L, Hallström A, Segersvärd S, Persson L, Ungerstedt U (1989) Dynamics of extracellular metabolites in the striatum after middle cerebral artery occlusion in the rat monitored by intracerebral microdialysis. J Cereb Blood Flow Metab 9: 607–616
15. Hillered L, Persson L, Bolander HG, Hallström A, Ungerstedt U (1988) Increased extracellular levels of ascorbate in the striatum after middle cerebral artery occlusion in the rat monitored by intracerebral microdialysis. Neurosci Lett 95: 286–290
16. Hillered L, Siesjö BK, Arfors K-E (1984) Mitochondrial response to transient forebrain ischemia and recirculation in the rat. J Cereb Blood Flow Metab 4: 438–446
17. Honegger CG, Langemann H, Krenger W, Kempf A (1989) Liquid chromatographic determination of common water-soluble antioxidants in biological samples. J Chromatogr 487: 463–468
18. Kaeser HE, Langemann H (1990) Oxygen free radicals and radical scavengers in neurology. In: Deecke L, Eccles JC et al (eds) From neuron to action: an appraisal of fundamental and clinical research. Springer, Berlin Heidelberg New York Tokyo, pp 557–563
19. Lancelot L, Callebert J, Revau M-L, Boulu RG, Plotkine M (1995) Hydroxyl radicals are not implicated in the necrosis induced by an intrastriatal perfusion of glutamate. J Cereb Blood Flow Metab 15: S86
20. Landolt H, Bullock R, Fujisawa H, McCulloch J, Miller S (1993) Glutamate diffusion characteristics determine neurotoxicity in the rat brain: 14C glutamate autoradiography. J Cereb Blood Flow Metab 13 [Suppl 1]: S753
21. Landolt H, Langemann H, Gratzl O (1993) On-line monitoring of cerebral pH by microdialysis. Neurosurgery 32: 1000–1004
22. Landolt H, Langemann H, Mendelowitsch A, Gratzl O (1994) Neurochemical monitoring and on-line pH measurements using brain microdialysis in patients in intensive care. Acta Neurochir (Wien) [Suppl] 60: 475–478
23. Landolt H, Lutz TW, Langemann H, Stauble D, Mendelowitsch A, Gratzl O, Honegger CG (1992) Extracellular antioxidants and amino acids in the cortex of the rat—monitoring by microdialysis of early ischemic changes. J Cereb Blood Flow Metab 12: 96–102
24. Langemann H, Mendelowitsch A, Landolt H, Alessandri B, Gratzl O (1995) Experimental and clinical monitoring of glucose by microdialysis. Clin Neurol Neurosurg 97: 149–155
25. Lyrer P, Landolt H, Kabiersch A, Langemann H, Kaeser H (1991) Levels of low molecular weight scavengers in the rat brain during focal ischemia. Brain Res 567: 317–320
26. Mangano RM, Schwarcz R (1983) Chronic infusion of endogenous excitatory amino acids into rat striatum and hippocampus. Brain Res Bull 10: 47–51
27. Nichols D, Attwell D (1990) The release and uptake of excitatory amino acids. Trends Pharm Sci 11: 462–468
28. Nilsson P, Hillered L, Pontén U, Ungerstedt U (1990) Changes in cortical extracellular levels of energy-related metabolites and amino acids following concussive brain injury in rats. J Cereb Blood Flow Metab 10: 631–637
29. Novelli A, Reilly JA, Lysko PG, Henneberry RC (1988) Glutamate becomes neurotoxic via the N-methyl-D-aspartate receptor when intracellular energy levels are reduced. Brain Res 451: 205–212
30. Schurr A, West CA, Rigor BM (1988) Lactate-supported synaptic function in the rat hippocampal slice prepartation. Science 240: 1326–1328
31. Shimada N, Graf R, Rosner G, Wakayama A, George CP, Heiss W-D (1989) Ischemic flow threshold for extracellular glutamate increase in cat cortex. J Cereb Blood Flow Metab 9: 603–606

32. Siesjö BK (1988) Mechanisms of ischemic brain damage. Crit Care Med 16: 954–963
33. Staub F, Baethmann A, Peters J, Weigt H, Kempski O (1990) Effects of lactacidosis on glial cell volume and viability. J Cereb Blood Flow Metab 10: 866–876
34. Swanson RA, Chen J, Graham SH (1994) Glucose can fuel glutamate uptake in ischemic brain. J Cereb Blood Flow Metab 14: 1–6
35. Takagi K, Ginsberg MD, Globus MYT, Dietrich WD, Martinez E, Kraydieb S, Busto R (1993) Changes in amino acid neurotransmitters and cerebral blood flow in the ischemic penumbral region following middle cerebral artery occlusion in the rat: Correlation with histopathology. J Cereb Blood Flow Metab 13: 575–585
36. Wu C (1994) Possible role of glutamatergic neurotransmission in regulating ethanol-evoked brain ascorbate release. Neurosci Lett 171: 105–108

Correspondence: B. Alessandri, Ph. D., Neurosurgical Laboratory, Department of Research, Kantonsspital, CH-4031 Basel, Switzerland.

Acta Neurochir (1996) [Suppl] 67: 13–20

Clinical Microdialysis: The Role of On-line Measurement and Quantitative Microdialysis

M.G. Boutelle* and **M. Fillenz**

Molecular Sensors Unit, University Laboratory of Physiology, Oxford, U.K.

Summary

The use of microdialysis in the clinic is examined in the light of lessons learnt from microdialysis in freely moving rats. Changes in concentrations of metabolites are an important index of the state of health of tissues. For effective therapeutic intervention rapid assays are essential. Enzyme-based on-line assays for glucose and lactate are described. By combining two of these assays simultaneous measurements of glucose and lactate, sampled at 2 min intervals can be obtained. The relation between dialysate concentrations and the true extracellular concentration of an analyte is dependent on conditions in the tissue sampled and cannot be calculated from in vitro probe recoveries. Furthermore, with acute implantation of the probe and possibly rapidly changing tissue conditions, there will be changes in probe recovery in vivo. Quantitative microdialysis allows the measurement of the true extracellular concentration and the probe recovery in vivo. The clinical applicability of a number of quantitative microdialysis methods is discussed, and three approaches highlighted. By increasing membrane length and reducing flow rate, recovery in vivo can be increased to 100%. In this case dialysate concentrations equal extracellular ones. By perfusing an inert exogenous compound an index of changes to extracellular volume and hence tissue oedema can be obtained. In the zero net flux method the infusion of a few concentrations of the analyte under study allows the direct determination of both the ECF concentration and the in vivo recovery. The latter can provide valuable information about changes in the physical as well as chemical state of the tissue. This can guide rapid effective therapeutic intervention.

Keywords: Clinical microdialysis; quantitative; enzyme-based assay.

Introduction

Microdialysis

Microdialysis has become established as a powerful sampling technique for neuroscience research and pharmacokinetic studies. It involves the implantation of a small segment of semipermeable membrane into the tissue to be studied. Subsequent slow perfusion with a solution matching the ionic composition of the extracellular fluid (ECF) allows species present in the tissue ECF to be carried across the membrane by the concentration gradient, and out of the microdialysis probe by the flow [1, 39]. Once collected, the microdialysate can be assayed using a wide range of chemical assays [27].

Clinical Microdialysis

There is now increasing interest in the possible use of microdialysis as an in situ clinical monitor. A number of experimental studies have been carried out in human subjects using microdialysis for transcutaneous and subcutaneous monitoring of low molecular compounds [10–12, 23]. These studies found that transcutaneous glucose was a good index of plasma glucose [11]. The measurement of lactate was more complicated. Transcutaneous lactate measurements also detected lactate concentration in sweat and subcutaneous lactate did not show a linear relation to plasma lactate since much of the lactate was of local origin [13]. In neonates there was a strong correlation between glucose dialysate levels and blood levels but there was also a correlation with neonate age, suggesting that diffusion of glucose to the probe is limited by the skin thickness [23].

Clinical applications of these techniques so far have been reports of the use of transcutaneous microdialysis of glucose and lactate in normal neonates [23] and one in premature neonates [9]. In the latter study there was

---

*Present address: Department of Chemistry, King's College Strand, London, U.K.

a strong relation between subcutaneous and blood glucose and a weak but highly significant relation between subcutaneous and plasma lactate.

There have also been reports in intensive care patients suffering from shock of the use of subcutaneous microdialysis [9, 13] and intravascular microdialysis [37]. In the latter study in addition to glucose and lactate, creatinine, urea, adenosine, inosine and hypoxanthine were assayed in the dialysate. Microdialysate values of all metabolites closely followed the changes in the corresponding blood samples. The in vivo recovery of the probe used was close to 100% and this approach therefore is a suitable method for continuous bedside monitoring of important metabolites in intensive care patients.

The possibility of brain microdialysis is of particular interest. The studies in the brain have been mainly concerned with the effects of trauma and stroke, typically the probe being introduced along with an intracranial pressure monitoring device. Concentrations of the energy related metabolites lactate, pyruvate and hypoxanthine were measured; the pyruvate/lactate ratio was found to be a particularly useful index [33]. The other group of compounds of considerable interest are the amino acids [34]. Such measurements have been combined with electrocorticographic recordings [8] or on-line pH measurements [24]. Correlations were found between levels of excitatory amino acids and high lactate/pyruvate ratios [33] and levels of amino acids and the onset of seizures [8].

The purpose of measurements in the clinic is to assess the level of neuronal damage, to see whether damage processes are continuing and to signal when there is a change in the tissue state which requires rapid therapeutic intervention. Thus indications of tissue ischaemia may be met by increasing cerebral perfusion pressure.

The aim of the present paper is to discuss how the lessons learnt from the extensive use of microdialysis in animals can be applied to microdialysis in the clinic.

We have used microdialysis in freely moving rats to study the delivery of energy substrates to neurones [16–18]. Neurones have a high rate of energy consumption and have no stores of energy. There is evidence that neurones in addition to glucose can also use lactate for energy production [14, 35]. Astrocytes, whose end feet surround cerebral capillaries, have a small store of glycogen with a rapid turnover [28]. There is now evidence from in vitro [32], in vivo [38] and clinical [15] work which suggests that astrocytes play some role in the supply of energy substrates for

neuronal metabolism. The extracellular concentration of glucose and lactate, which can be detected using microdialysis, is the balance between supply and utilisation processes. Deviations from normal extracellular concentrations of glucose and/or lactate therefore may reflect pathological changes in neuronal metabolism in cerebral blood flow or in astrocyte function. Monitoring the extracellular concentration of glucose and its metabolic products is therefore of considerable interest in clinical practice.

Requirements

Initial clinical microdialysis measurements attempted to assay as many compounds as possible, since it was not known which would be the most useful index of pathological changes. From this work the significance of certain substances is now emerging. These include glucose, lactate and pyruvate. Ratios of two of these have proved to have prognostic value. For effective therapeutic interventions it is essential to detect changes rapidly. This requires reliable, rapid on-line systems. We have developed a sensitive enzyme-based on-line assay for use with animals that can be adapted for clinical measurement of two compounds simultaneously.

The relation between levels of compounds in the microdialysate and their concentration in the brain extracellular fluid is determined not only by the microdialysis probe; properties of the tissue sampled also play a role. True extracellular concentrations can be determined using quantitative microdialysis. Furthermore this approach can provide additional valuable information about the state of the tissue as well as processes of supply and removal of the compounds under investigation.

Methods

On-line Assay System

We have designed an assay system which is sensitive enough and fast enough to allow rapid on-line sampling [4, 5]. This avoids chromatographic separation and hence slower sampling because of column elution times. It is also important that the assays be stable, share common components and be simple to use. Enzymes can be used very effectively to react with a target analyte. They are very specific for their substrate, giving good selectivity; subsequent regeneration of the enzyme can be arranged to produce a mediator molecule which can be detected electrochemically, giving good sensitivity. We have developed a series of enzyme reactors which can assay microdialysate on-line. For stability the enzymes are covalently immobilised onto silica beads and packed into a rugged bed. For the selective detection of glucose, lactate or glutamate we have used the oxidase enzymes glucose oxidase, lactate oxidase or glutamate oxidase. These enzymes are stable (being of extracellular origin), fast and have stable bound cofactors. The hydrogen peroxide produced then reacts with a second enzyme and a component of the buffer to give a species which is detected highly efficiently at a downstream electrode to give a single current peak proportional to the sample content. Full experimental details for the construction and use of the enzyme bed have been published previously [4, 5].

To operate on-line, the microdialysate continuously flows into a sample loop of an injector valve. After a chosen volume has been collected, the microdialysate is automatically injected for analysis into the buffer stream normally flowing through the enzyme reactor. The valve then resets itself to collect the next sample. The system inherently rejects interference from species present in the brain, and hence the dialysate, which can be oxidised by the electrode. As further protection against interference from electroactive species we also pre-oxidise the microdialysate using an on-line tubular electrode system [3]. This also provides an invaluable dialysate flow meter giving an instantaneous warning of any interference with flow such as twisting or disconnection of the tubes.

Assay for Glucose

A typical calibration response for glucose is shown in Fig. 1A. The glucose assay has a detection limit of < 20 pmol injected on column and a linear response up to 2 mM glucose (with 5 μL injections), which covers dialysate levels and injection volumes likely to be encountered in the clinic (Fig. 1B). A 10% variation in this response was found over 50 days' use. In our animal experiments we assay dialysate from the brains of freely moving rats at 2.5 min intervals.

Assay for Lactate

The lactate assay gives a very fast response peak with a detection limit of < 7 pmol on column. It has a linear response up to approximately 250 μM before showing the Michaelis-Menten curvature of the lactate oxidase (Fig. 1C). In our animal studies and in clinical use dialysate levels may be expected to exceed this. This problem is overcome by restricting the volume injected onto the column; thus all likely levels can be kept within the linear range of the assay. In addition, volume restriction improves the time resolution of the assay. With freely moving rats, this assay is also used at 2.5 min sampling.

Simultaneous Assay for Glucose and Lactate

Preliminary clinical data has suggested that the ratio of glucose and lactate levels is a better therapeutic index than the level of either of the compounds alone. However, because both enzyme beds give the same signal to the electrode it is not possible to use them in series. We have now designed a new on-line injector component which will use a 10 port valve to split the dialysate between two sample loops, and hence allow the injection of dialysate on-line onto two assay systems running in parallel. The proposed experimental set-up is shown in Fig. 2. The dialysate flows through the two injection loops sequentially. The lactate assay has the highest sensitivity and can saturate if too much lactate is injected on-column. Consequently, this assay is connected to the smaller first loop. The glucose assay will be connected to the second loop. The resultant system is capable of assay of both glucose and lactate on-line with an improved sampling interval of 2 min.

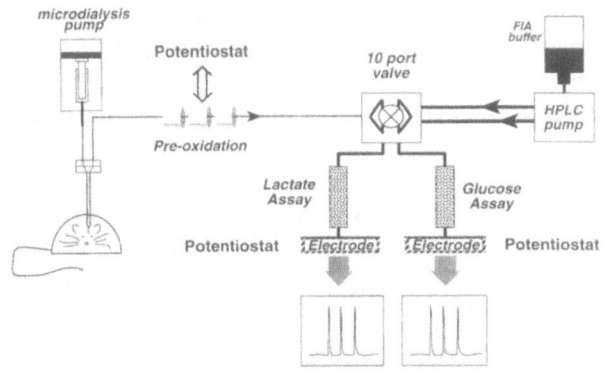

Fig. 2. Experimental set-up for simultaneous on-line monitoring of glucose and lactate

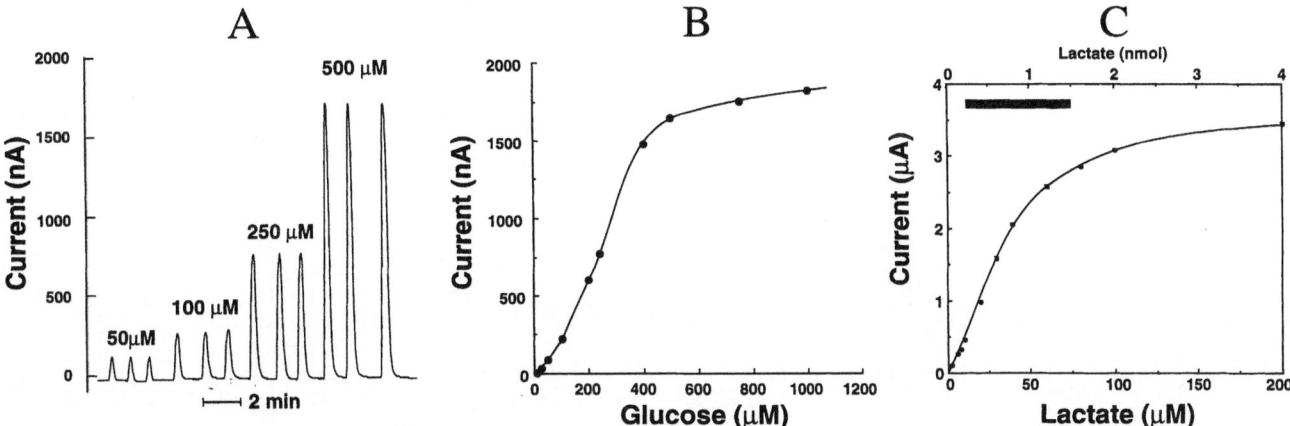

Fig. 1. (A) Flow injection response of glucose assay to injection of glucose standards. (B) Calibration curve for glucose assay. Each point represents mean ± sem (n = 5). Error bars are the size of the points or smaller. (C) Calibration curve for lactate assay. Each point represents mean ± sem (n = 5). Error bars are the size of the points or smaller. The lower x-axis shows lactate concentration, the upper x-axis shows lactate content injected on column. The black bar indicates the range of basal and stimulated lactate contents of 5 μL microdialysate samples

Difference Between Dialysate and ECF Concentrations

The true extracellular concentration of a compound cannot be derived simply from the properties of the probe determined in vitro, since the additional factors dependent on the tissue play a role in determining in the relationship between dialysate concentration and ECF concentration [2, 7, 30].

With a probe placed in a beaker containing a well-stirred solution of a substance, the drop in concentration is across the membrane of the probe and so determines the relationship between the concentration in the dialysate and the concentration in the beaker; this is the *recovery* or *extraction fraction* of the probe in vitro (Fig. 3A). The in vitro recovery is constant for a given flow rate, temperature and probe type.

In contrast, for a dialysis probe implanted in tissue, sampling an exogenous substance, the drop in concentration occurs mainly across the tissue (Fig. 3B). The reason for this is that in vivo the substance must diffuse along a tortuous path around the cells, and the cells themselves represent an excluded volume from which no substance can come. Transport across the tissue now limits supply of substance to the probe and the *recovery* or *extraction fraction in vivo* is much lower than that found in vitro. Furthermore, the in vivo recovery is now not constant for a given probe but dependant on a tissue property—the extracellular volume.

Additional factors come into play in the case of a dialysis probe implanted in tissue sampling a substance actively supplied and removed from the ECF by the tissue either by release, transport or metabolism [7,

30]. In this case, which applies to all compounds of clinical interest, the in vivo recovery and hence the dialysate concentration for a given flow rate and probe type, depends on the extracellular volume and the rates of the active processes. In the tissue close to the probe these active processes respond to the concentration gradient across the tissue by either increasing their rate of supply or decreasing their rate of removal (Fig. 3C). This has the effect of steepening the concentration gradient, increasing the supply of substance to the probe and hence increasing the probe *recovery* or *extraction fraction in vivo* compared to that for an exogenous compound. This is shown on Fig. 3C for turnover rates of 10, 100, 1000. As the rate of the active processes increases so the in vivo recovery increases (and the volume of tissue required to support the loss of substance to the probe decreases). In the limit of infinitely fast rates the curve becomes identical with Fig. 3A, hence the in vitro recovery should represent the upper limit for the in vivo recovery. Bungay has shown that an exception to this is exocytotic release of neurotransmitters, whose rate is not directly affected by a change in local ECF concentration caused by the probe [6].

Quantitative Microdialysis

As the relationship between dialysate concentration and ECF concentration is complex, various methods have been developed in animal experiments to approach this problem. They can be grouped into two types: setting in vivo recovery to 100%, and varying a parameter to measure the in vivo recovery.

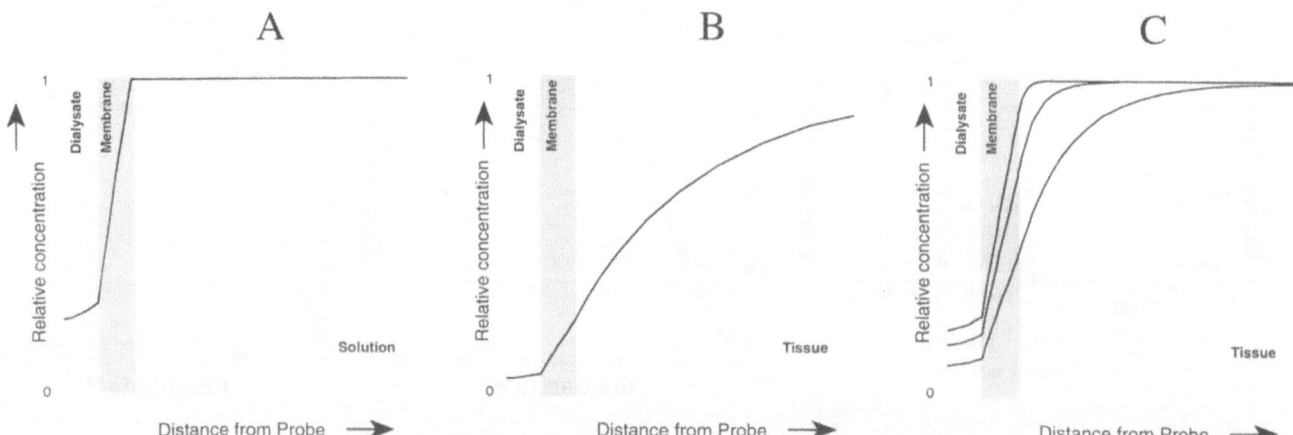

Fig. 3. Schematic concentration profiles to a microdialysis probe. (A) In vitro. (B) Implanted in vivo for a passively distributed exogenous compound. (C) Implanted in vivo for an endogenous compound which is supplied, uptaken and metabolised by the tissue. Increasing steepness in the curves represents an increase by a factor of ten in the tissue handling rates. The distance in the tissue represents about 200 µm

Setting in vivo Recovery to 100%

The central concept behind these approaches is that when in vivo recovery is 100% the dialysate concentration equals the ECF concentration.

Lerma [25] has achieved 100% recovery by recirculating dialysate through a conventional probe. He has then used this method to measure the ECF levels of glutamate in the anaesthetised rat. Clinically this method has been used for subcutaneous monitoring of glucose [36]. A problem for the clinical use of this method is its poor time resolution (several hours per sample) and the practical difficulties of switching from the recirculation mode to the extraction mode to assay the sample.

Another approach is to alter the microdialysis conditions to achieve near 100% recovery. This can be done by increasing the active membrane length, decreasing the probe diameter and slowing the flow rate. Hillered and Ungerstedt have recently used this approach in clinical studies [37]. Preliminary results suggest that a concentric probe with a 10 mm active membrane at a flow rate of 0.3 µL/min achieves near 100% recovery. The advantage of this strategy is that it is simple to implement reliably, as it requires no separate in vivo measurement. However, the conditions for 100% recovery in normal tissue *may no longer apply* during acute traumatic episodes. This can be checked by measurement *in vivo* for a given probe type by seeing whether dialysate concentration remain unchanged by a decrease in flow rate. This approach is also limited by the length of membrane that can be accommodated by a given tissue.

Measurement of in vivo Recovery

As the in vivo recovery depends on the state of the tissue both physically (e.g. ECF volume) and functionally (e.g. rates of supply and removal), measurement of the in vivo recovery has the advantage that additional information about the state of the tissue is obtained and so provides a further clinical use of microdialysis.

Loss of Labelled Compound

As diffusion across the dialysis membrane is symmetrical in both directions it is possible to add to the perfusate a known level of an identifiable compound and then monitor the loss to the brain by measuring the level in the dialysate. If a compound is exogenous such as sucrose then only the passive (physical) aspects of in vivo recovery are taken into account. This could pro-vide a clinical method for monitoring any ECF volume changes caused for example by oedema. However, such values do not help with the measurement of a particular endogenous species. In animal studies this has been overcome by adding tracer quantities of the desired analyte which have a radiolabel, to distinguish the infused chemical from that found in the tissue [20]. It seems very unlikely that such an approach would be acceptable clinically.

Variation of Flow

An alternative approach is the variation of flow. Microdialysis is performed at a number of different flow rates including very low flow rates. Jakobson has described a simple graphical analysis which calculates the ECF concentration and hence the in vivo recovery [21]. The method works by extrapolating from low flow rates to the 100% recovery which would be achieved at zero flow. Whilst a change in flow rate is simple to implement there are many practical problems associated with very low flow rates (0.1 µL/min and slower). These include the time taken for a measurement, handling low volumes and evaporative loss.

Zero Net Flux

The zero net flux method was first described by Lönnroth for human subcutaneous measurement of glucose [26]. The approach is outlined in Fig. 4. The basis of the method is to find the concentration of infused substance which neither loses to the brain nor

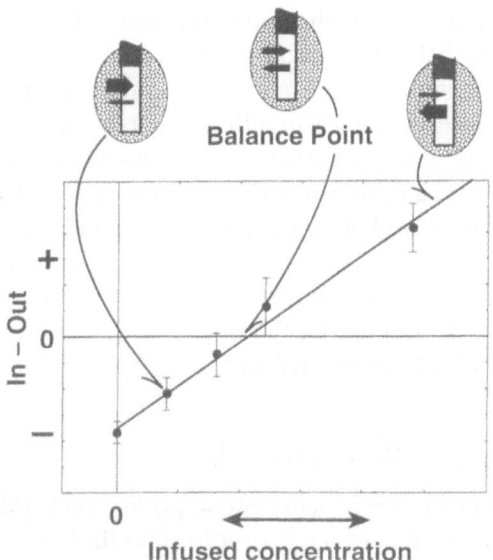

Fig. 4. Principle of the zero net flux method

gains from it when passed through the dialysis probe. As there is no net flux across the membrane this concentration must equal the true ECF concentration. In practice a small number (3–5) of infused concentrations are chosen, a plot of gain or loss against this concentration made and the ECF concentration determined by regression. The gradient of the plot is the in vivo recovery. In rats Justice has used this method for dopamine [22], and has shown that the level is not affected by the extraction of other neurochemicals during microdialysis [41]. We have used it to determine ECF levels for glucose [17] glutamate [29] and lactate. The importance of the method is that it makes no assumptions about the tissue sampled. Values for the ECF concentration and the in vivo recovery are measurements.

A graphical approach can be used to examine how changes in different brain tissue properties can alter microdialysate levels by changing true ECF levels and by changing the in vivo recovery.

Interactions Between the Tissue and Microdialysis

Tissue Processes Affecting ECF Levels

Simplest case is the effect of tissue processes on ECF levels. The ECF level of a substance is determined by the balance between all the release processes and all the uptake processes. If the release rate is increased (by physiological activation or pathological change) it will temporarily outstrip the uptake rates and a new balance will be found at a higher ECF concentration. In Fig. 5 this can be seen to be equivalent to a parallel shift of the in vivo recovery line along the x-axis. Consequently, the dialysate concentration increases by the same proportion. Similarly, a decrease in release rates or an increase in uptake or utilisation rates causes removal processes to outstrip supply leading to a fall in ECF and hence a proportionate fall in dialysate levels. All early animal work with microdialysis assumed that this was how microdialysis worked with a constant in vivo recovery. As discussed above, this is in fact only true in all circumstances for the special case of dialysis probes with 100% in vivo recoveries.

Tissue Processes Affecting in vivo Recovery

It is also possible for changes in supply and removal processes, and the state of the tissue to affect the in vivo recovery, and hence the slope of graphs such as Figs. 4 and 5.

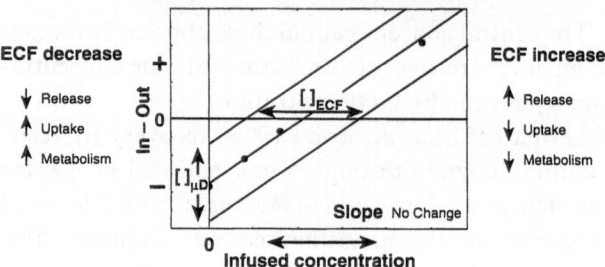

Fig. 5. Effects of tissue processes on extracellular concentration [ ]$_{ECF}$ and dialysate concentration [ ]$_{\mu D}$

Passive Processes

If the extracellular volume increases, it is easier for compounds to diffuse around the cells to the probe, the concentration gradient shown in Fig. 3B becomes steeper, the dialysate concentration increases, and hence the in vivo recovery increases. As the ECF concentration does not change this is shown on Fig. 6 by an increase in slope, pivoting about the ECF concentration. Such an increase in ECF volume could be caused clinically by vasogenic oedema. Similarly, a decrease in extracellular volume leads to a reduction in dialysate concentration, and a decrease in in vivo recovery. This is shown on Fig. 6 by a decrease in slope pivoting about the unchanged ECF concentration. Such a decrease in ECF volume could be caused by excitotoxic oedema. In both cases the dialysate concentration does NOT reflect the extracellular level.

Active Processes

Figure 3C demonstrates that rates of supply and removal of compound by the tissue affect the delivery of substance to the probe and hence the dialysate

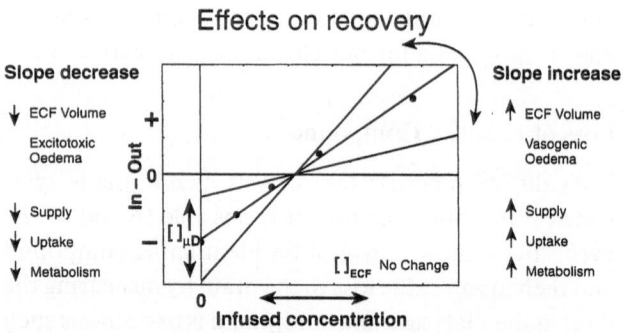

Fig. 6. Effects of tissue processes on in vivo recovery (slope) and dialysate concentration [ ]$_{\mu D}$

concentration and the in vivo recovery. Supply processes which will alter the slope include physiological ones, such as transporter mechanisms (but not exocytotic release), and pathological ones such as loss of releasing neurones or astrocytes or a change in the permeability of the blood brain barrier due to repair or vasogenic oedema [40]. Removal processes which will alter the slope include uptake carriers and intracellular and extracellular metabolism. Figure 6 shows the direction of these effects.

A comparison with Fig. 5 emphasises an important difference between the effects on ECF concentration and the effects on in vivo recovery. Supply and removal processes act in opposition on ECF concentrations but in concert on the in vivo recovery. In many situations this means that a change in both supply and removal will affect both the ECF concentration and the in vivo recovery, but may move in opposite directions and have a different time course. We have found such effects during the local application of veratridine on glucose levels in the rat [19]. However, if there is a matched change in supply and removal the ECF concentration will remain unaffected but the slope of Fig. 6 will change pivoting about the ECF concentration. In this case the dialysate level does not reflect the ECF concentration. This has been found for dopamine in the rat nucleus accumbens following a 6-OH-dopamine lesion [31], but clearly such a situation is also possible following physiologically induced changes, or pathological events such as spreading depression or following stroke.

The Role of Quantitative Microdialysis in the Clinic

In animal microdialysis, measuring neurotransmitters, quantitative approaches are not routinely used. This is because changes in exocytotic neurotransmitter release do not affect in vivo recovery, it is assumed that changes in active uptake processes are small and mainly affect the ECF concentration (equivalent to the movements shown diagramatically in Fig. 5) and conditions are chosen to minimise physical changes to the tissue during the microdialysis experiment. With these assumptions dialysate levels can be taken as a good index of ECF levels.

In clinical microdialysis the situation is more complicated. Firstly, the tissue is unlikely to be in a stable state. Measurements are initially made immediately after probe implantation when the blood brain barrier may be compromised. Furthermore, during the measurement the extracellular volume can be altered by vasogenic and excitotoxic oedema. Secondly, the tissue

supply and removal processes may undergo large changes. This could be caused by spreading depression following probe placement, local failure of energy supply due to infarction, or massive stimulation of neuronal energy requirements due to excitotoxic overflow from a nearby infarct. The effects of such changes on microdialysate levels will be of the type shown in Fig. 6, where the principal effect is on in vivo recovery and there is a decoupling between microdialysate and ECF levels. Quantitative microdialysis can help control these situations and provide information about them in the following ways:

(a) The simplest approach is to use probe lengths and flow rates which allow 100% recovery in vivo. In this case the dialysate concentrations equal those in the ECF and are not altered by changes in the tissue. It is important that the 100% recovery is not compromised, but this could be checked by a temporary decrease in flow rate which should not alter the dialysate concentration. (b) The permanent addition of a known low level of an inert exogenous compound (such as sucrose) to the perfusate together with measurement of dialysate levels of this compound would allow changes in the extracellular volume to be measured. Such an approach would provide a rapid monitor for vasogenic and excitotoxic oedema. (c) Using a variant of the zero net flux method both the ECF concentration and the in vivo recovery could be measured. A simple version of the method would be to automatically switch between two perfusate solutions: one containing a known concentration of analyte; the other containing no analyte. On-line measurement of dialysate levels and simple processing of the data by a computer would give a real-time display of both the ECF concentration and the in vivo recovery. The latter would be an index of both passive and active changes in the tissue state.

In conclusion, rapid on-line assays and quantitative microdialysis can provide important additional information in the clinic which can guide on-going therapeutic intervention.

Acknowledgements

We would like to thank Dr. Peter Bungay of the National Institutes of Health USA for extensive discussions and help with the construction of Fig. 3. We acknowledge the financial support of SERC (UK) and EPSRC (UK).

References

1. Benveniste H (1989) Brain microdialysis. J Neurochem 52: 1667–1679
2. Benveniste H, Hansen AJ (1991) Practical aspects of using

microdialysis for detemination of brain interstitial concentrations. In: Robinson TE et al (eds) Microdialysis in the neurosciences. Elsevier, Amsterdam, pp 81–100

3. Berners MOM, Boutelle MG, Fillenz M (1994) On-line measurement of brain glutamate with an enzyme/polymer- coated tubular electrode. Anal Chem 66: 2017–2021

4. Boutelle M, Fray A, Fellows L, Berners M, Miele M, Fillenz M (1994) Biosensors for on-line analysis of microdialysate-flow injection analysis using ferrocene mediated enzyme packed beds. In: Louilot A et al (eds) Monitoring molecules in neuroscience -94, pp 37–38

5. Boutelle MG, Fellows LK, Cook C (1992) Enzyme packed bed system for on-line measurement of glucose, glutamate, and lactate in brain microdialysate. Anal Chem 64: 1790–1794

6. Bungay P (1995) Personal communication

7. Bungay PM, Morrison PF, Dedrick LD (1990) Steady-state theory for quantitative microdialysis of solutes and water in vivo and in vitro. Life Sci 46: 105–119

8. Carlson H, RonneEngstrom E, Ungerstedt U, Hillered L (1992) Seizure related elevations of extracellular amino acids in human focal epilepsy. Neurosci Lett 140: 30–32

9. De Boer J, Korf J, Plijter Groendijk H (1994) In vivo monitoring of lactate and glucose with microdialysis and enzyme reactors in intensive care medicine. Int J Artif Organs 17: 163–170

10. De Boer J, PlijterGroendijk H, Korf J (1992) Continuous monitoring of glucose with a transcutaneous microdialysis probe (6). Lancet 340: 547–548

11. De Boer J, PlijterGroendijk H, Korf J (1993) Microdialysis probe for transcutaneous monitoring of ethanol and glucose in humans. J Appl Phys 75: 2825–2830

12. De Boer J, PlijterGroendijk H, Visser KR, Mook GA, Korf J (1994) Continuous monitoring of lactate during exercise in humans using subcutaneous and transcutaneous microdialysis. Eur J Appl Physiol 69: 281–286

13. De Boer J, Potthoff H, Mulder POM, Dofferhoff ASM, Van TRJ, PlijterGroendijk H, Korf J (1994) Lactate monitoring with subcutaneous microdialysis in patients with shock: a pilot study. Circ Shock 43: 57–63

14. Dringen R, Gebhardt R, Hamprecht B (1993) Glycogen in astrocytes: possible function as lactate supply for neighboring cells. Brain Res 623: 208–214

15. Eyre J, Struart A, Forsyth R, Heaviside D, Bartlett K (1994) Glucose export from the brain in man: evidence for a role for astrocytic glycogen as a reservoir of glucose for neural metabolism. Brain Res 635: 349–352

16. Fellows LK, Boutelle MG (1993) Rapid changes in extracellular glucose levels and blood flow in the striatum of the freely moving rat. Brain Res 604: 225–231

17. Fellows LK, Boutelle MG, Fillenz M (1992) Extracellular brain glucose levels reflect local neuronal activity: a microdialysis study in awake, freely-moving rats. J Neurochem 59: 2141–2147

18. Fellows LK, Boutelle MG, Fillenz M (1993) Physiological stimulation increases non-oxidative glucose metabolism in the brain of the freely moving rat. J Neurochem 60: 1258–1263

19. Fray A, Fillenz M (1995) Veratridine changes in vivo recovery of glucose in rat striatum. Brain Res Assoc Abstr 12: 71

20. Jacobson 1, Hamberger A (1984) Veratridine-induced release in vivo and in vitro of amino-acids in the rabbit olfactory-bulb. Brain Res 299: 103–112

21. Jacobson I, Sanberg M, Hamberger A (1985) Mass transfer in brain dialysis devices-a new method for the estimation of extracellular amino acids concentration. J Neurosci Methods 15: 263–268

22. Justice JB (1993) Quantitative microdialysis of neurotransmitters. J Neurosci Methods 48: 263–276

23. Korf J, De BJ, Baarsma R, Venema K, Okken A (1993) Monitoring of glucose and lactate using microdialysis: applications in neonates and rat brain. Dev Neurosci 15: 240–246

24. Landolt H, Langemann H, Mendelowitsch A, Gratzl O (1994) Neurochemical monitoring and on-line pH measurements using brain microdialysis in patients in intensive care In: Ito U et al (eds) Brain edema IX. Acta Neurochir [Suppl] 60: 475–478 (Wien)

25. Lerma J, Herranz AS, Herreras O, Abraira B, Rio RMD (1986) In vivo determination of extracellular concentration of amino acids in the rat hippocampus. A method based on brain dialysis and computerized analysis. Brain Res 384: 145–155

26. Lonnroth P, Jansson P-A, Smith U (1987) A microdialysis method allowing characterization of intercellular water space in humans. Am J Physiol 253: E228–E231

27. Lunte CE, Scott DO, Kissinger PT (1991) Sampling living systems using microdialysis probes. Anal Chem 63: A 773

28. Magistretti PJ, Sorg O, Martin J-L (1993) Regulation of glycogen metabolism in astrocytes: physiological, pharmacological, and pathological aspects. In: Murphy S et al (eds) Astrocytes. Academic Press, San Diego, pp 243–265

29. Miele M, Berners M, Boutelle M, Kusakaba H, Fillenz M (1996) The determination of the extracellular concentration of glutamate using quantitative microdialysis. Brain Res 707: 131–133

30. Morrison PF, Bungay PM, Hsiao JK, Mefford IN, Dykstra KH, Dedrick RL (1991) Quantitative microdialysis. In: Robinson TE, et al (eds) Microdialysis in the neurosciences. Elsevier, Amsterdam, pp 47–80

31. Parsons LH, Smith AD, Justice JB (1991) The in vivo microdialysis recovery of dopamine is altered independently of basal level by 6-hydroxydopamine lesions to the nucleus- accumbens. J Neurosci Methods 40: 139–147

32. Pellerin L, Magistretti P (1994) Glutamate uptake into astrocytes stimulates aerobic glycolysis: a mechanism coupling neuronal activity to glucose utilisation. Proc Natl Acad Sci USA 91: 10625–10629

33. Persson L, Hillered L (1992) Chemical monitoring of neurosurgical intensive care patients using intracerebral microdialysis. J Neurosurg 76: 72–80

34. RonneEngstrom E, Hillered L, Flink R, Spannare B, Ungerstedt U, Carlson H (1992) Intracerebral microdialysis of extracellular amino acids in the human epileptic focus. J Cereb Blood Flow Metab 12: 873–876

35. Schurr A, West CA, Rigor BM (1988) Lactate-supported synaptic function in the rat hippocampal slice preparation. Science 240: 1326–1328

36. Sternberg F, Meyerhoff C, Mennel C, Hoss U, Mayer H, Bischof F, Pfeiffer EF (1994) Calibration problems of subcutaneous glucosensors when applied 'in-situ' in man. Horm Metab Res 26: 523–525

37. Stjernstrom H, Karlsson T, Ungerstedt U, Hillered L (1993) Chemical monitoring of intensive care patients using intravenous microdialysis. Intensive Care Med 19: 423–428

38. Swanson R (1992) Physiologic coupling of glial glycogen metabolism to neuronal activity in brain. Can J Physiol Pharmacol 70: S138–S144

39. Ungerstedt U (1986) Microdialysis—a new bioanalytical sampling technique. Current Separations 7: 43–46

40. Westergren I, Nyström B, Hamberger A, Johansson B (1994) Amino acids in extracellular fluid in vasogenic edema. In: Ito U et al (eds) Brain edema. Acta Neurochir (Wien) [Suppl] 60: 124–127

41. Sam PM, Justice JB (1996) Effect of general microdialysis induced depletion on extracellular dopamine. Anal Chem 68: 724–728

Correspondence: Martyn G. Boutelle, Ph.D, Department of Chemistry, King's College, Strand, London, WCZR 2LS, U.K.

Acta Neurochir (1996) [Suppl] 67: 21–23
© Springer-Verlag 1996

Intracerebral Microdialysis Markedly Inhibits the Propagation of Cortical Spreading Depression

T.P. Obrenovitch and **E. Zilkha**

Department of Neurological Surgery, Institute of Neurology, London, U.K.

Summary

It is accepted that the ionic composition of the medium perfused through a microdialysis probe should match that of the extracellular fluid (ECF) under physiological conditions. In contrast, the possibility that control artificial cerebrospinal fluid may influence the experimental or pathological conditions under study, by buffering changes in the ECF composition, has been neglected. Spreading depression (SD) is a propagating transient suppression of electrical activity due to cellular depolarization which may contribute to neuronal damage in focal ischaemia, and underlie the migraine aura. Here we report that microdialysis markedly inhibits SD propagation, by buffering the sudden increase in extracellular K^+ associated with this event. This effect is independent of the microdialysis flow rate and does not result from tissue injury following probe implantation. This finding clearly illustrates that microdialysis can influence the pathological conditions under investigation.

Keywords: Microdialysis; spreading depression; cerebral ischaemia; epilepsia.

Introduction

Microdialysis is a versatile sampling technique which requires implantation of a dialysis fibre through which an artificial medium is perfused [1]. It is generally acknowledged that the composition of the perfusion medium should match that of the ECF under physiological conditions [2]. In contrast, the possibility that the perfusion of control artificial CSF (ACSF) may buffer critical changes in the ECF composition, produced by the conditions under study, has been overlooked. Here, we report that microdialysis inhibits the propagation of spreading depression (SD) by buffering the transient increase in extracellular K^+ associated with this phenomenon.

Methods and Material

Rats were anaesthetised with halothane throughout the experiment. SD was elicited by application of 160 mM K^+ through a microdialysis probe implanted in the cerebral cortex, i.e. the perfusion medium was switched for 5 min from control ACSF to a solution containing 160 mM K^+ and 25 mM Na^+ (liquid switch CMA/110; CMA/Microdialysis, Stockholm, Sweden). Propagating SD, identified as a transient negative shift of the extracellular direct current (DC) potential, was recorded 2 to 3 mm posteriorly from the triggering site, either with a chlorided silver electrode placed in the inlet tubing of a microdialysis probe (Fig. 1) [6, 7] or with a chlorided silver wire identical in size to a dialysis fibre (i.e. 250 μ o.d. and 2 mm in length). The 'microdialysis electrode' made it possible to record SD propagation as the ECF composition surrounding the dialysis membrane was altered. A delay of 2 h post-implantation allowed the preparation to stabilize.

The effect of microdialysis on SD propagation was examined in a first series, by comparing the SD-induced DC potential negative shift recorded with microdialysis electrodes perfused at 1 μl/min, with that obtained with chlorided silver wires. As these experiments demonstrated a strong inhibition of SD propagation by microdialysis, a second series aimed to examine whether this effect was dependent on the microdialysis flow rate. Five consecutive SDs were elicited, with each SD followed by 20 min of recovery. Control ACSF in the recording microdialysis probe was either stagnant throughout (no flow) or flowing at: 0.25, 0.5, 1.0, and 2.0 μl/min. The flow was changed 10 min before SD elicitation whenever necessary. Suspecting that microdialysis inhibition of SD propagation was due to control ACSF in the probe buffering transient changes in the ECF composition, we then tested whether increasing the concentration of K^+ in the perfusion medium would restore SD propagation. We used 30 and 60 mM K^+-ACSF because it has been repeatedly shown that extracellular K^+ reaches these levels during SD [4, 5]. The perfusion medium of the recording probe was modified for 10 min, starting 3 min before the application of high K^+ at the frontal site to trigger SD. Each SD elicitation was followed by 20 min of recovery during which control ACSF was perfused.

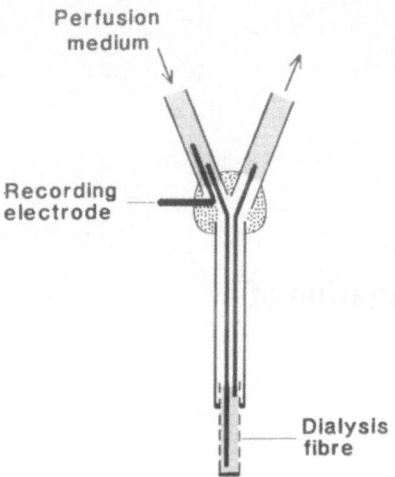

Fig. 1. Schematic representation of the recording microdialysis probes, incorporating a chlorided silver electrode in the inlet tubing, which made it possible to record the extracellular DC potential as the composition of the ECF surrounding the dialysis membrane was altered. The potential recorded between the microdialysis electrode and a reference electrode placed under the scalp is equivalent to that obtained with a glass capillary electrode whose tip is positioned next to the outer surface of the dialysis membrane [6]

Results

With 250 μ o.d. bare chlorided silver wires, propagating SD was recorded as a transient DC potential negative shift of 8.2 ± 0.8 mV, n = 7. This amplitude, around half that of SD recorded with conventional glass capillary electrodes, was further reduced when the recording electrode was incorporated within a microdialysis probe perfused with normal ACSF (3.5 ± 0.4 mV, n = 10; $P < 0.001$, Student's t test) (Fig. 2).

The amplitude of the first SD, recorded with microdialysis electrodes and stagnant ACSF, was 5.9 ± 0.4 mV (n = 13), i.e. still markedly reduced in comparison with those recorded with chlorided silver

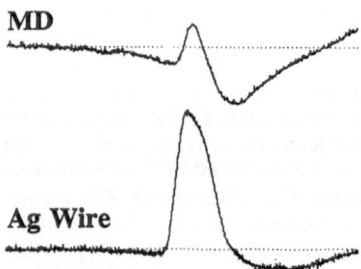

Fig. 2. Representative inhibition of propagating SD by microdialysis. Only a small shift of the DC potential remained when the signal was recorded through a microdialysis probe perfused with control ACSF (*MD*). SD was much larger when it was recorded with a bare chlorided silver wire, identical in size to the dialysis fibre (*Ag Wire*)

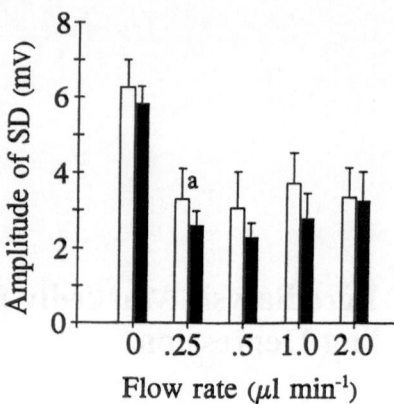

Fig. 3. Effect of microdialysis flow rate on propagating SD recorded with a microdialysis electrode. Five SDs were triggered 2–3 mm frontal from the recording probe. In the control group, ACSF was stagnant throughout (Open columns; n = 6). In the other, the rate of perfusion was as indicated below the x-axis (solid columns; n = 7). Data are mean $\pm$ SEM. [a]$P < 0.002$, comparison with the first SD by Student's paired t test

wires. Incremental increases of the perfusion flow rate to 2 μl/min did not reduce further the magnitude of subsequent SDs (Fig. 3). Perfusion of the recording microdialysis probe with a medium containing 30 mM K^+ was sufficient to produce a marked increase in the amplitude of the DC shift characteristic of SD (8.2 ± 0.8 mV, n = 7; $P < 0.001$ for comparison with perfusion with control ACSF by Student's paired t test). Sixty mM K^+ further increased SD amplitude (12.0 ± 0.5 mV, n = 7; $P < 0.001$). Parallel experiments showed that, alone, 30–60 mM K^+ in the perfusion medium does not trigger SD (data not shown).

Discussion

These results demonstrate that microdialysis markedly inhibits the propagation of spreading depression (Fig. 2), presumably by buffering the transient increase in ECF K^+ which is associated with this event [8]. They further showed that this inhibition was independent of the microdialysis flow rate. The pool of stagnant ACSF within the microdialysis probe, by itself, was sufficient to buffer markedly transient changes in the surrounding ECF composition (Fig. 3). Microdialysis had previously been suspected to inhibit SD propagation. With glass microelectrodes placed 0.5 mm from a dialysis probe, Fabricius and co-workers [3] observed a major DC shift during only 25% of the SD episodes. This effect explains the difficulties experienced in previous attempts to demonstrate glutamate efflux associated with propagating SD using microdialysis [3, 10], whereas marked glutamate release was recorded with local application of high K^+ through the microdialysis probe [12].

The inhibition of SD propagation by microdialysis clearly points to a critical pitfall of this method: i.e. potential influence on the experimental or pathological conditions under investigation, by buffering transient changes in the ECF composition. This critical pitfall is likely to apply to a number of conditions. Imposing low K^+ levels in the brain cells microenvironment may be particularly deleterious because extracellular K^+ content is the main determinant of the cellular membrane potential, and it influences markedly both neuronal interaction and excitability [9, 11]. Epileptic seizures and the ischaemic penumbra are two important situations that may be prone to such a detrimental interaction of microdialysis. Buffering ACSF strongly may also interfere with such conditions by reducing acidosis in the tissue surrounding the microdialysis fibre.

References

1. Benveniste H, Hüttemeier PC (1990) Microdialysis-theory and application. Prog Neurobiol 35: 195–215
2. De-Boer P, Damsma G, Fibiger HC, Timmerman W, De Vries JB, Westerink BHC (1990) Dopaminergic-cholinergic interactions in the striatum: the critical significance of calcium concentrations in brain microdialysis. Naunyn Schmiedebergs Arch Pharmacol 342: 528–534
3. Fabricius M, Jensen LH, Lauritzen M (1993) Microdialysis of interstitial amino acids during spreading depression and anoxic depolarization in rat neocortex. Brain Res 612: 61–69
4. Hansen AJ, Zeuthen T (1981) Extracellular ion concentrations during spreading depression and ischemia in rat brain cortex. Acta Physiol Scand 113: 437–445
5. Kraig RP, Nicholson C (1978) Extracellular ionic variations during spreading depression. Neuroscience 3: 1045–1059
6. Obrenovitch TP, Richards DA, Sarna GS, Symon L (1993) Combined intracerebral microdialysis and electrophysiological recording: methodology and applications. J Neurosci Methods 47: 139–145
7. Obrenovitch TP, Urenjak J, Zilkha E (1994) Intracerebral microdialysis combined with recording of extracellular field potential: a novel method for investigation of depolarizing drugs in vivo. Br J Pharmacol 113: 1295–1302
8. Obrenovitch TP, Zilkha E (1995) High extracellular potassium, and not extracellular glutamate, is required for the propagation of spreading depression. J Neurophysiol 3: 2107–2114
9. Rutecki PA, Lebeda FJ, Johnston D (1985) Epileptiform activity induced by changes in extracellular potassium in hippocampus. J Neurophysiol 5: 1363–1373
10. Scheller D, Heister U, Kolb J, Tegtmeier F (1993) On the role of excitatory amino acids during generation and propagation of spreading depressions. In: Lemenkühler A et al (eds) Migraine: basic mechanisms and treatments. Urban and Schwarzenberg, Munich, pp 355–366
11. Spira ME, Yarom Y, Zeldes D (1984) Neuronal interactions mediated by neurally evoked changes in the extracellular potassium concentration. J Exp Biol 112: 179–197
12. Wahl F, Obrenovitch TP, Hardy AM, Plotkine M, Boulu R, Symon L (1994) Extracellular glutamate during focal cerebral ischaemia in rats: time course and calcium dependency. J Neurochem 63: 1003–1011

Correspondence: Tihomir P. Obrenovitch, Ph.D, Department of Neurological Surgery, Institute of Neurology, Queen Square, WC1N 3BG, London, U.K.

Acta Neurochir (1996) [Suppl] 67: 24–27
© Springer-Verlag 1996

Delayed Neuronal Damage Following Focal Ischemic Injury in Stroke-Prone Spontaneously Hypertensive Rats

K. Shima, **T. Shirotani**, and **H. Chigasaki**

Department of Neurosurgery, National Defense Medical College, Tokorozawa, Saitama, Japan

Summary

We detected the delayed accumulation of ^{45}Ca in the lateral part of the striatum 3 days after distal middle cerebral artery (MCA) occlusion in stroke-prone spontaneously hypertensive rats (SHRSP). However, the mechanism of delayed neuronal damage in the striatum, which is not supplied by the occluded MCA, remains unknown. The aim of this study was to evaluate whether the delayed damage involves alterations in the extracellular release of neurotransmitter monoamines and amino acids. Chronological changes in the distribution of neuronal damage were determined by ^{45}Ca autoradiography. The microdialysis probes were inserted into either the medial or lateral part of the striatum. The dialysate content of monoamines, their metabolites and amino acids was determined by analytical techniques.

^{45}Ca accumulation was detected only in the cortex and corpus callosum by 24 hours postischemia, and extended to the pyramidal tract, thalamus and lateral portion of the striatum by 3 days. A 3-fold increase in glutamate content, and a 2-fold increase in dopamine content were observed only in the lateral part of the striatum following ischemia.

The results suggest that excessive release of glutamate and dopamine is related to delayed neuronal damage that occurs in the lateral part of the striatum in this ischemic model.

Keywords: Cerebral ischemia; striatum; glutamate; microdialysis.

Introduction

The striatum is highly vulnerable to ischemia. It also is innervated richly by both the corticostriatal glutamatergic pathway and by nigrostriatal dopaminergic projections, which have been shown to interact with each other [2]. Excitatory amino acids, such as glutamate, may contribute to ischemic cell death, by causing an intracellular overload of calcium [3]. It has been suggested that dopamine contributes to ischemic cell death by producing oxygen radicals [5], or by potentiating the excitotoxic effects of glutamate [8].

It has been demonstrated that distal occlusion of the striate branches of the middle cerebral artery (MCA) resulted in a reproducible focal infarction in stroke-prone spontaneous hypertensive rats (SHRSP), but not in normotensive rats [4, 17]. The infarct produced by this procedure was limited to the ipsilateral cerebral cortex and did not extend to the basal ganglia. Recently, we have detected the delayed accumulation of ^{45}Ca in the non-ischemic remote areas after focal ischemia in SHRSP [18]. Furthermore, we found a hyperemia after 4 hours of MCA occlusion in the lateral part of the striatum, in which the accumulation of ^{45}Ca was detected at 3 days postischemia [9]. The mechanism of delayed neuronal damage in the striatum remains unexplained. In our previous study, MK-801, an N-methyl-D-aspartate (NMDA) antagonist, significantly reduced the neuronal damage in the striatum [18]. We therefore speculated that this phenomenon in the striatum may be regulated by the interactions of a variety of neurotransmitters. The aim of this study was to evaluate whether the delayed damage involves alterations in the extracellular release of neurotransmitter monoamines and amino acids.

Materials and Methods

Male SHRSP, 11 to 14 weeks old and weighing 250 to 350 g, were used. Following intubation, the animals were ventilated artificially with a mixture of 70% N_2, 30% O_2, and 1%–1.5% halothane. Rectal temperature was kept at 37°C with a heating lamp. The right MCA was occluded through a retroorbital burr-hole craniectomy using an operating microscope. The occlusion was distal to the striate branches of the MCA and 0.7–1 mm dorsal to the rhinal fissure [4, 17].

^{45}Ca Autoradiography

Experiments were performed as described previously [6, 18]. Briefly, following 4 h, 24 h, 3 days, 7 days, and 14 days of MCA occlusion, $^{45}CaCl_2$ (3.7 MBq/100 g body weight; New England Nuclear) was injected intravenously. Five hours after the injection, the rats were decapitated. Then the brains were quickly removed, frozen and cut into 20 μm-thick sections for autoradiographic studies.

Microdialysis Procedures

The microdialysis probe (outer diameter 0.22 mm; membrane length 3 mm; molecular weight cut-off, 50000; BDP-I-8-03, EICOM, Kyoto) was inserted into either the medial (n = 14) or lateral (n = 14) part of the right striatum. The co-ordinates were 0.5 mm anterior, 3 mm lateral to the bregma, and 3.5 mm ventral from the brain surface in the medial side group, and 0.5 mm anterior, 4.5 mm lateral to the bregma, and 2.8 mm ventral from the brain surface in the lateral side group. The dialysis probes were continuously perfused at 2 μl/min with Ringer's solution. The body temperature, blood pressure and arterial blood gases were maintained in the normal range throughout the experiment.

After a 3-hour period for stabilization of the baseline, the right MCA was occluded. The dialysate samples were collected every 20 min until 2 hours after MCA occlusion. Two hours after the occlusion, the rats were sacrificed and each probe position verified. The animals were randomly divided into two groups, one (n = 7) for the measurement of monoamines and their metabolites and the other (n = 7) for the measurement of amino acids. The dialysate concentrations of monoamines and their metabolites included dopamine (DA), dihydroxyphenilacetic acid (DOPAC), homovanillic acid (HVA), and 5-hydroxyindole-3-acetic acid (5-HIAA) were determined by high-performance liquid chromatography (HPLC) with an electrochemical detector (ECD-100, EICOM). The dialysate concentrations of amino acids included glutamate (Glu), taurine (Tau), alanine (Ala), glutamine (Gln), and γ-aminobutyric acid (GABA) were analysed by HPLC with electrochemical detection following precolumn derivatization with o-phthaldialdehyde.

Statistical Analysis

Data are expressed as means ± SD. Differences were assessed by analysis of variance, followed by Dunnett's test or the Student's t-test.

Results

^{45}Ca accumulation was detected only in the cortex at 4 h and 24 h post-ischemia, and extended to the pyramidal tract, thalamus and the lateral part of the striatum by 3 days. After 7 and 14 days, the regional ^{45}Ca became more prominent (Fig. 1).

Following MCA occlusion, extracellular Glu and DA levels were significantly (p < 0.01) increased in the lateral part of the striatum, while there were no significant changes in the medial part of the striatum (Figs. 2 and 3). The Glu level had returned to baseline values by 60 min after the occlusion. The GABA and Tau levels were also significantly increased only in the

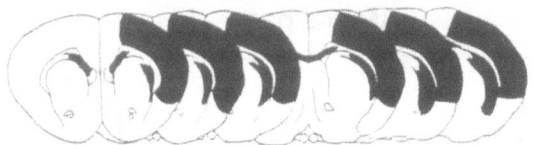

Fig. 1. Schematic diagram of accumulation of ^{45}Ca 7 days following MCA occlusion. Coronal sections are shown at the level of the striatum. ^{45}Ca accumulated in the cerebral cortex, corpus callusum and the lateral part of the striatum

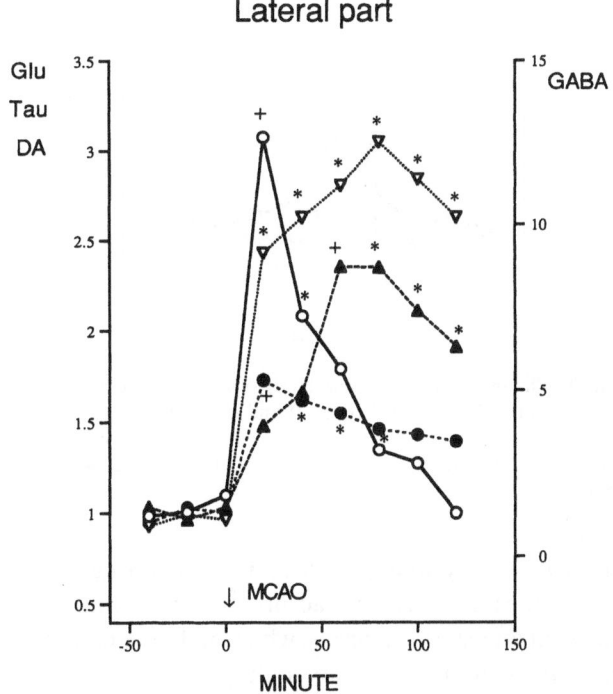

Fig. 2. Changes in the dialysate levels of glutamate (Glu), taurine (Tau), γ-aminobutyric acid (GABA) and dopamine (DA) sampled from the lateral part of the striatum, expressed as times basal level. *p < 0.05, +p < 0.01 vs. preischemic value (Dunnett's test). MCAO middle cerebral artery occlusion, ○ Glu, ▽ Tau, ● GABA, ▲ DA

lateral part of the striatum. However, Gln and Ala levels remained at their baseline values.

Discussion

It is well documented that postischemic calcium accumulation is time-dependent and coincident with the progression of ischemic injury [6]. Using a focal ischemic model in which infarction is limited to the cerebral cortex, we found that ^{45}Ca accumulated not only in the cerebral cortex, but also in the corpus callosum, ipsilateral pyramidal tract, the ventral posterior nucleus of the thalamus, and the lateral part of the striatum, which is not supplied by the occluded MCA [18]. It is assumed that ^{45}Ca had accumulated in

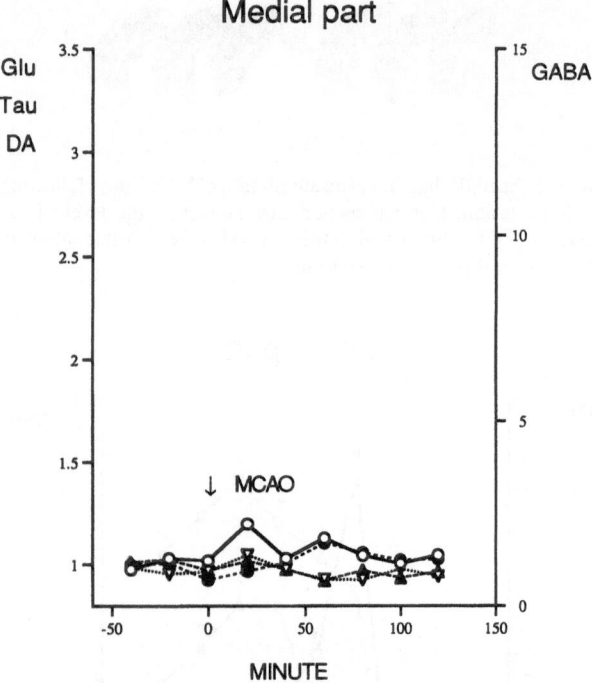

Medial part

Fig. 3. Changes in the dialysate levels of glutamate (*Glu*), taurine (*Tau*), γ-aminobutyric acid (*GABA*) and dopamine (*DA*) sampled from the medial part of the striatum, expressed as times basal level. *MCAO* middle cerebral artery occlusion. ○ Glu, ▽ Tau, ● GABA, ▲ DA

the irreversibly injured cell and degenerating axons [1]. In the thalamus, ^{45}Ca accumulation was limited to the ventroposterior nucleus, which had fiber connnections in anatomic proximity to the postcentral gyrus of the cerebral cortex. The delayed ischemic damage in this area may result from retrograde degeneration following thalamo-cortical fiber damage caused by the precedent ischemic insult to the postcentral gyrus [13]. The damage in the pyramidal tract and corpus callosum may also be caused by anterograde degeneration resulting from ischemic cortical injury. However, the mechanism of delayed neuronal damage in the lateral part of the striatum remains unexplained. In our previous study using the same MCA occlusion model, the lateral part of the striatum showed a significant increase in local cerebral blood flow and decrease in local glucose metabolism 4 hours after ischemia [9]. This flow-metabolic uncoupling is assumed to be luxury perfusion. The lateral part of the striatum has a cortico-striatal glutamatergic pathway [11]. Glutamate induces a release of a diffusible messenger with strikingly similar properties to endothelium-derived relaxing factor (EDRF) released from endothelial cells in response to vasodilators [7]. Hyperemia of the lateral striatum may be caused by EDRF because

glutamate is released in cortical ischemic areas. We have shown that MK-801 significantly reduced the neuronal damaged volume in the striatum as well as in the cortex and thalamus [18]. These findings are highly suggestive of the role of glutamate in the neuronal damage in the striatum. The results of our microdialysis study demonstrate that focal cortical injury is associated with different neurotransmitter changes in the medial and lateral parts of the striatum. Significant increases in the extracellular concentrations of Glu, Tau, GABA and DA were observed only in the lateral striatum, where the infarct area did not extend until 24 hours after MCA occlusion. Glu attained its peak level after 20 min of ischemia and then rapidly declined to baseline. Sensory and motor areas project topographically onto the dorsolateral striatum [11], and were affected by ischemia in the present model [18]. It is suggested that neuronal depolarization may occur in the cerebral cortex, causing a release of Glu stored in vesicles. Perschak and Cuenod [16] have observed that Glu and Asp were significantly increased in the striatum following a 4-min stimulation of the ipsilateral frontal cortex. It follows that spiky Glu release could be detected only in the lateral striatum. Increased concentrations of Tau [12], GABA [15] and DA [10] could be an indirect response to Glu activation of specific receptors. It can thus be speculated that a massive release of these neurotransmitters may occur at axon terminals of the striatum inducing neuronal damage. On the other hand, the lateral striatum is adjacent to the ischemic regions, and ischemic brain edema may contribute to the changes observed in this area [14].

In conclusion, the present results indicate that focal cortical ischemia in SHRSP is associated with different neurotransmitter changes in the medial and lateral parts of the striatum. In addition, the results suggest that the postischemic delayed neuronal damage in the lateral striatum may have been caused by massive Glu release, together with the DA release.

References

1. Benveniste H, Huttemeier PC, Johansen FF, Diemer NH (1989) Calcium 45 accumulation in the dentate hilus: possible effect of NMDA receptors blockers. In: Hartmann A, Kuschinsky W (eds) Cerebral ischemia and calcium. Springer, Berlin Heidelberg New York Tokyo, pp 266–273
2. Cheramy A, Romo R, Godeheu G, Baruch P, Glowinski J (1986) In vivo presynaptic control of dopamine release in the cat caudate nucleus: II. Facilitatory or inhibitory influence of L-glutamate. Neuroscience 19: 1081–1090
3. Choi DW (1987) Ion dependence of glutamate neurotoxicity. J Neurosci 7: 369–379

4. Coyle P, Jolainen PT (1983) Differential outcome to middle cerebral artery occlusion in spontaneously hypertensive stroke-prone rats (SHRSP) and Wistar Kyoto (WKY) rats. Stroke 14: 605–611

5. Damsma G, Boisvert DP, Mudrick LA, Wenkstern D, Fibiger HC (1990) Effect of transient forebrain ischemia and pargyline on extracellular concentrations of dopamine, serotonin, and their metabolites in the rat striatum as determined by in vivo microdialysis. J Neurochem 54: 801–808

6. Dienel GA (1984) Regional accumulation of calcium in postischemic rat brain. J Neurochem 43: 913–925

7. Garthwaite J, Charles SL, Chees-Williams R (1988) Endothelium-derived relaxing factor release on activation of NMDA receptors suggests role as an intercellular messenger in the brain. Nature 336: 385–388

8. Globus MY-T, Busto R, Dietrich WD, Martinez E, Valdes I, Ginsberg MD (1988) Intra-ischemic extracellular release of dopamine and glutamate is associated with striatal vulnerability to ischemia. Neurosci Lett 91: 36–40

9. Kita H, Shima K, Tastumi M, Chigasaki H (1995) Cerebral blood flow and glucose metabolism of ischemic rim in middle cerebral artery-occluded spontaneously hypertensive stroke-prone rats. J Cereb Blood Flow Metab; 15: 235–241

10. Leviel V, Gobert A, Guibert B (1990) The glutamate-mediated release of dopamine in the rat striatum: further characterization of the dural excitatory-inhibitory function. Neuroscience 39: 305–312

11. McGeorge AJ, Faull RLM (1989) The organization of the projection from the cerebral cortex to the striatum in the rat. Neuroscience 29: 503–537

12. Menendez N, Herreras O, Solis JM, Herranz AS, del Rio MR (1985) Extracellular taurine increase in rat hippocampus evoked by specific glutamate receptor activation is related to the excitatory potency of glutamate agonists. Neurosci Lett 102: 64–69

13. Nagasawa H, Kogure K (1990) Exo-focal postischemic neuronal death in the rat brain. Brain Res 524: 196–202

14. Nordborg C, Sokrab TEO, Johansson BB (1991) The relationship between plasma protein extravasation and remote tissue changes after experimental brain infaction. Acta Neuropathol (Berl) 82: 118–126

15. Perouansky M, Grantyn R (1990) Is GABA release modulated by presynaptic excitatory amino acid receptors? Neurosci Lett 113: 292–297

16. Perschak H, Cuenod M (1990) In vivo release of endogeneous glutamate and aspartate in the rat striatum during stimulation of the cortex. Neuroscience 35: 283–287

17. Shima K, Umezawa H, Chigasaki H, Okuyama S, Araki H (1994) Local cerebral blood flow and glucose metabolism in chronic focal ischaemia of stroke-prone spontaneously hypertensive rats. Neurological Res 16: 289–296

18. Shirotani T, Shima K, Iwata M, Kita H, Chigasaki H (1994) Calcium accumulation following middle cerebral artery occlusion in stroke-prone spontaneously hypertensive rats. J Cereb Blood Flow Metab 14: 831–836

Correspondence: Katsuji Shima, M.D., Department of Neurosurgery, National Defense Medical College, 3-2 Namiki, Tokorozawa, Saitama 359, Japan.

Acta Neurochir (1996) [Suppl] 67: 28–30

The Measurement of Extracellular Inorganic Phosphate Gives a More Reliable Indication for Severe Impairment of Cerebral Cell Function and Cell Death than the Measurement of Extracellular Lactate

D. Scheller, J. Kolb, U. Peters, and F. Tegtmeier

Janssen Research Foundation, Neuss, Federal Republic of Germany

Summary

The measurement of cerebral extracellular lactate levels has been suggested to be used to monitor cerebral function in intensive care. However, although an increase of extracellular lactate levels is a sensitive parameter for increased cellular activity in general, it will be shown that its prognostic value is limited in regard to the severity of the impairment of cellular function. As an alternative, the measurement of the extracellular levels of inorganic phosphate (IP) or adenosine is proposed here: Whereas extracellular lactate levels increased rapidly to about the same extents during ischemia (IS) and spreading depression (SD), IP rose during IS only. Adenosine, on the other hand, increased during both events to a different degree. If, therefore, lactate was the only parameter to be monitored after a cerebral insult, the results would not allow to discriminate between a transient, spontaneously recovering event as a SD and a long-lasting or an irreversible loss of cell function as in persisting ischemia/hypoxia. The measurement of IP, therefore, seems to be more suitable than that of lactate or adenosine since IP will appear within the extracellular space only after a sustained failure of membrane function. Thus, the measurement of IP changes turned out to be the more useful parameter for intensive care supervision.

Keywords: Spreading depression; ischemia; cerebral microdialysis; intensive care monitoring; inorganic phosphate; adenosine; lactate.

Introduction

Lactate has been shown to be released during spreading depression (SD) and cerebral ischemia (IS) and has been proposed as an indicator for metabolic disturbances of brain function [4, 5, 7, 9, 11]. However, inorganic phosphate (IP)—primarily derived from ATP dephosphorylation—also can leak out of the cells under such conditions [8]. Since adenosine is produced too under these circumstances, it also might leak into the extracellular space (ECS) [10]. Thus, IP and/or adenosine might be useful parameters for monitoring the brain energy status and thus could be used as an indicator for the possible recovery of the function. The present study, therefore, was performed to determine and to compare the extracellular changes of inorganic phosphate, adenosine and lactate by means of the microdialysis technique. SD and IS were chosen as pathological events. During SD, the loss of membrane function is transient in contrast to persisting during IS where the membrane failure is irreversible [1–3, 6].

Methods

Male Wistar rats of 230 to 260 g were anaesthetized with urethane (1.5 to 2 g/kg) and a microdialysis (MD) probe (perfusate: artificial CSF, flow rate: 2 µl/min) was inserted into the cortex (coordinates: $-2/2$ AP/ML to the bregma). Within the immediate vicinity, a microelectrode (ME) for direct current (DC) recordings was inserted. SD was induced by switching the perfusate from CSF to a high K-CSF (120 mM) for 2 min. Ischemia was induced by cardiac arrest (0.3 ml saturated $MgCl_2$ i.v.). Inorganic phosphate was determined photometrically [8]. Lactate was determined by HPLC analysis [9]. Adenosine was determined by HPLC after derivatisation with chloroacetaldehyde [12].

Results

Dialysate IP concentration did not change during SD. However, it increased about 2-fold 30 to 60 minutes after the occurrence of SD and then returned to basal levels. During IS, IP rapidly increased 9.3-fold. The rise started subsequent to the anoxic DC-depolarisation (Figs. 1–3).

Dialysate lactate concentration rose 2.6-fold during SD and returned to basal levels within about 45 min. During IS, lactate increased 2.6-fold starting to rise

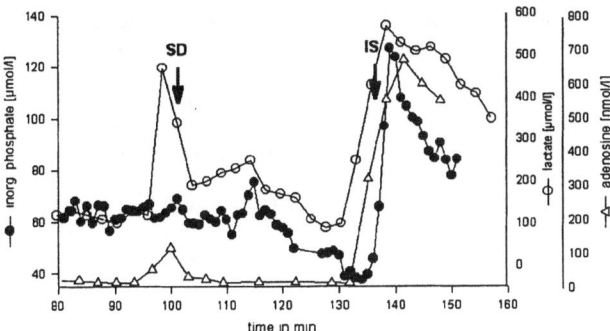

Fig. 1. Concentration changes of lactate, phosphate and adenosine in dialysate fractions during spreading depression and ischemia. Time courses of the parameters from single experiments are combined

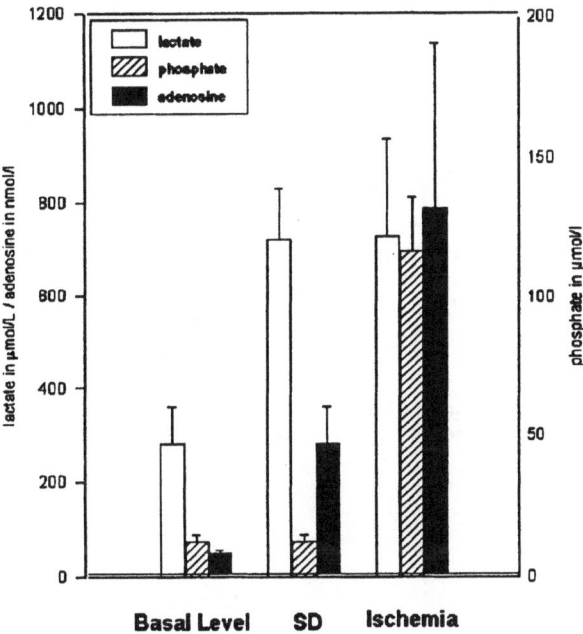

Fig. 2. Basal levels and maximal concentration changes of lactate, phosphate and adenosine in dialysate fractions during spreading depression and ischemia

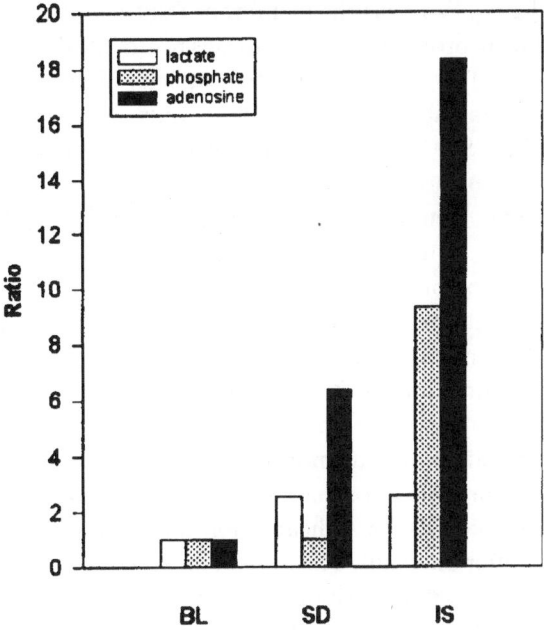

Fig. 3. Changes of the maximal concentrations of lactate, phosphate and adenosine during spreading depression and ischemia in relation to basal levels (*BL*)

Discussion

In the initial phase of ischemia, anaerobic glycolysis is maximally stimulated [11]. The dialysate lactate levels rise about 2.6-fold. During SD, the increase of lactate is about the same (Fig. 3). Thus, the anaerobic glycolysis seems to be maximally stimulated during both events. In contrast, extracellular adenosine levels differ markedly under both circumstances (Fig. 3). The extracellular rise of adenosine is less pronounced during SD than during IS. Since ATP is completely degraded during complete ischemia [11], the extracellular levels of adenosine seem to be a direct indicator for the catabolism subsequent to the membrane failure and its equilibration between ICS and ECS. The lower levels of adenosine during SD, however, seem to be a consequence of the new steady state between ATP consumption and delivery. The changes of adenosine, therefore, may indicate regulatory activities of the cells occurring via adenosine transporters [13]. In contrast to lactate and adenosine, inorganic phosphate appears within the ECS during IS only (Fig. 3) although it could be expected to appear there during SD too in conjunction with adenosine release.

Ischemia and spreading depression are accompanied by a negative DC shift of 15 to 25 mV [1–3, 6]. The negative DC shift has been interpreted as an indication for membrane depolarization and loss of ion homeo-

immediately after onset of ischemia and prior to anoxic depolarisation. After some time, dialysate lactate tended to decrease although the ischemia persisted (Figs. 1–3).

Dialysate adenosine concentration increased 6.4-fold during SD and returned to basal levels within 30 to 40 min. During IS, dialysate adenosine concentration started to rise immediately after onset of ischemia and continued to rise to levels 18.3-fold its normal levels (Figs. 1–3).

stasis [2, 3]. Whereas the membrane failure is irreversible during prolonged IS, it is always reversible during SD [2, 3]. This indicates that the capacity of the cells and their membranes to keep functioning during an insult like SD is maintained, otherwise a recovery would not be possible.

Whereas lactate and adenosine start to rise with onset of IS, inorganic phosphate appears in the ECS after the membranes have been depolarised [8]. This indicates that phosphate seems to appear in the ECS only if membrane failure persists for a prolonged period of time and/or is irreversible. Thus, inorganic phosphate appears within the ECS under conditions of severe impairment of membrane function. The appearance of inorganic phosphate in the ECS can presumably be taken as an indicator for the "point of no return" after an insult. The measurement of IP, therefore, is more suitable to monitor intensive care patients during or after conditions of cerebral ischemia than to measure lactate or adenosine.

References

1. Bures J, Buresova O, Krivanek J (1974) The mechanism and applications of Laos spreading depression of electroencephalographic activity. Academic Press, New York
2. Caspers H, Speckmann EJ, Lehmenkühler A (1987) DC Potentials of the cerebral cortex: seizure sctivity and changes in gas pressures. Rev Physiol Biochem Pharmacol 106: 127–178
3. Hansen AJ (1985) Effect of anoxia on ion distribution in the brain. Physiol Rev 65: 101–148
4. Kuhr WG, Korf J (1988) N-methyl-D-aspartate receptor involvement in lactate production following ischemia or convulsion in rats. Eur J Pharmacol 155: 145–149
5. Lauritzen M, Hansen AJ, Kronborg D, Wieloch T (1990) Cortical spreading depression is associated with arachidonic acid accumulation and preservation of energy charge. J Cereb Blood Flow Metab 10: 115–122
6. Nicholson C, Kraig RP (1981) The behaviour of extracellular ions during spreading depression. In: Zeuthen T (ed) The application of ion-selective microelectrodes. Elsevier, Amsterdam, pp 217–238
7. Scheller D, Kolb J (1991) The internal reference technique in microdialysis: a practical approach to monitoring dialysis efficiency and to calculating tissue concentrations from dialysis samples. J Neurosci Methods 40: 31–38
8. Scheller D, Kolb J, Tegtmeier F, Lehmenkühler A (1992) Extracellular changes of inorganic phosphate are different during spreading depression and global cerebral ischemia of rats. Neurosci Lett 141: 269–272
9. Scheller D, Kolb J, Tegtmeier F (1992) Lactate and pH change in close correlation in the extracellular space of the rat brain during cortical spreading depression. Neurosci Lett 135: 83–86
10. Sciotti VM, Van Wylen DGL (1993) Attenuation of ischemia-induced extracellular adenosine accumulation by homocystein. J Cereb Blood Flow Metab 13: 208–213
11. Siesjö BK (1978) Brain energy metabolism. Wiley, New York
12. Svensson JO, Jonzon B (1990) Determination of adenosine and cyclic adenosine monophosphate in urine using solid-phase extraction and high-performance liquid chromatography with fluorometric detection. J Chromatogr 529: 437–441
13. Van Belle H (1993) Adenosine promoters: an overview of existing strategies. Current Opin Invest Drugs 2: 1191–1199

Correspondence: D. Scheller, M.D., Janssen Research Foundation, Raiffeisenstr. 8, D-41470 Neuss, Federal Republic Germany.

Acta Neurochir (1996) [Suppl] 67: 31–36

A Concept for the Introduction of Cerebral Microdialysis in Neurointensive Care

H. Landolt[1], **H. Langemann**[2], and **B. Alessandri**[2]

[1]Neurosurgical Clinic, Kantonsspital, Aarau, and [2]Neurosurgical Laboratory, Department of Research, Basel, Switzerland

Summary

Before microdialysis (MD) can be introduced into the clinic as an improved method of cerebral monitoring, certain ethical, methodological and clinical factors must be considered. Access to the brain for probe insertion is offered by craniotomy or by routine intracranial pressure (ICP) monitoring and the additional lesion is minimal. Care must be taken that the two devices do not interfere with each other. In contrast to ICP monitoring, MD provides information about multiple aspects of brain metabolism. We can monitor either still intact tissue to prevent additional damage, or injured brain to decide on and control therapies. The parameters used must reflect pathological changes at an early stage, and the analysis should be available on-line or immediately after sample collection. The effects of factors such as tube length and flow rate on the behaviour of the chosen parameters (in our case on-line pH, radical scavengers and uric acid) in the MD set-up must be investigated in vitro and in animal models before use in the clinic. The range of non-pathological values of parameters of interest in human brain should be known. For this purpose we took measurements during an extracranial-intracranial bypass operation, and were able to compare values with those in a severely damaged brain. The mutual chronology of parameter changes and clinical events must be clear. Future aspects include the use of low-flow methods offering nearly 100% recovery, improved analytical methods, and combination of MD with other monitoring methods to obtain more exact information.

Keywords: Microdialysis; brain metabolism; intensive care; methodology.

Introduction

Our main reason for getting additional information from the brain of patients during neurointensive care is to detect and prevent secondary cerebral lesions, which remain a challenge in spite of continued progress in management of head trauma [4]. An improvement in monitoring methods could help to avoid them or treat them at a time early enough to be really effective.

Much of our knowledge of normal and pathological brain metabolism has been obtained from animal experiments and has not yet been modified for clinical use. Cerebral monitoring with microdialysis (MD) provides access in the patient to many of the biochemical parameters used in experimental neurobiology. MD has advantages over other monitoring methods, such as measurements of intracranial pressure (ICP), electroencephalogram (EEG), O_2 level in tissue and jugular venous oxygen saturation, because it supplies continuous neurochemical information directly from the extracellular space of the cortex. The feasibility of this bedside method has been shown by different authors [10, 12, 15] and intraoperative use has provided preliminary knowledge of basal and pathological values, e.g., during brain tumour resection [6], extra-intracranial bypass operations or aneurysm operations [13].

Surgical access to the human brain can be gained during routine ICP monitoring or craniotomy, permitting the insertion of a probe into the brain tissue both ethically and practically. One advantage of MD is that it potentially provides information about multiple biochemical parameters at the same time, whereas ICP measurement can tell us only about one physical parameter (and by calculation about cerebral perfusion pressure). Additionally left-over dialysate can be used to investigate other aspects (e.g., pharmacokinetics [14]).

However, the introduction of monitoring with cerebral MD demands careful planning of the concept and of the ethical aspects. The aim in our clinic was to use an ischaemia-sensitive parameter which could be measured bedside, therefore we developed the on-line pH meter [9]. Other parameters, namely glucose and lactate to detect disturbances in energy metabolism [12] and oxygen radical scavengers such as ascorbic acid (Asc), glutathione (GSH), cysteine (Cys) [11] together with uric acid (UA) were also included. We describe here some in vitro and in vivo experiments which we made to assess the reliability and feasibility of these parameters before their use in the clinic. The first measurements of some of these parameters in patients are also reported.

Methods

In vitro and in vivo Experiments

a) On-line pH meter in vitro. The measured pH of the dialysate depends partly on the relative recoveries of bicarbonate and carbondioxide (CO_2), the major buffer substances in the extracellular fluid. These recoveries were measured at various flow rates (0.5–7.5 µl/min) at 38 °C by a previously described method [9], using a constant tube length of 30 cm between the probe exit and the pH cell. Additionally, the effects of varying this tube length (2–45 cm) on the recovery of CO_2 was investigated at a constant flow rate of 2 µl/min.

b) On-line pH in vivo. Microdialysis probes (CMA/10, 3 mm membrane, 0.5 mm diameter, tube length 30 cm) were inserted into the parietal cortex of 2 spontaneous hypertensive rats under general anaesthesia (Halothane 0.5%–1.0% in O_2). The probes were perfused with 0.9% saline and on-line pH of the dialysate was measured at different flow rates (0.5–5µl/min) [9].

c) The relative recovery rates of GSH and Cys were measured in vitro at room temperature (flow rate 2 µl/min, probe CMA/10, 3 mm membrane). The perfusion medium was Ringer solution (Na^+ 155 mM, K^+ 4mM, Ca^{2+} 2.75mM, HCO_3-1mM, Cl^- 164.5mM, pH 7.1). The concentrations of GSH and Cys in the outer medium were between 2.5 µM and 20 µM, a range comparable to that found in vivo in the spontaneous hypertensive rat before and after middle cerebral artery occlusion [11]. GSH and Cys were analysed using reverse phase HPLC with electrochemical detection [7].

d) Probes were sterilized at 60 °C with ethylene dioxide before use in patients. To check the sterility and permeability of the probes for bacteria were perfused 3 sterilised probes (CMA/20, 4 mm membrane, 0.5 mm diameter) with a suspension of staphylococcus aureus Wood 46 (10^6 bacteria/ml) during 24 h. Afterwards the tips of the probes were stuck into sterile Agar-culture plates, which were then incubated and checked for contamination.

Measurements in Patients

The probe (CMA/20, 4mm membrane, 0.5 mm diameter) was implanted into the cortex through a 2 mm incision of the dura during the neurosurgical procedure. Perfusion with sterile 0.9% normal saline was started before implantation, at a flow rate of 2 µl/min. Fractions were collected every 30 or 60 min, the samples being frozen at −80 °C as soon as possible, Asc, UA, Cys and GSH were determined in the dialysates (20 µl) using HPLC with electrochemical detection [7].

In patient 1, the probe was implanted during a protective extracranial-intracranial bypass operation. The patient did not show any neurological deficits before or after the operation. Samples were collected during 2 h, to try to measure leavels in minimally damaged brain. Patient 2 had a severe head injury caused by a fall. The MD probe was implanted during the operation for evacuation of a subdural haematoma. Cranial perfusion pressure was only 31–41 mm Hg, so that there was severely reduced cerebral perfusion. Samples were collected for 8 h, flow rate being reduced to 1 µl/min for 2h, in an

attempt to assess basal levels [8]. The patient died a few hours after the end of measurement.

Results

In vitro and in vivo Experiments

a) The effects of changing of flow rate on in vitro recovery of bicarbonate and CO_2, as measured in the on-line pH meter, are shown in Fig. 1a. Bicarbonate recovery was generally lower than that of CO_2 (exception, 0.5 µl/min). For bicarbonate, recovery decreased as expected as the flow rate was increased. However, there was an anomaly in the recovery of CO_2; recovery increased between 0.5 µl and 2 µl, decreasing afterwards with increasing flow. Recovery of CO_2 was also markedly and inversely dependent on the length of the tubing between the probe and the flow-through cell (Fig. 1b).

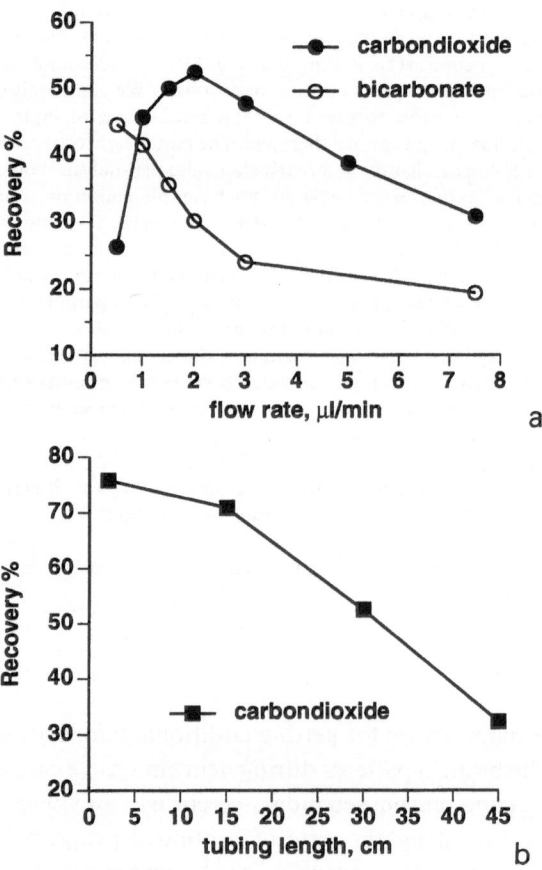

Fig. 1. (a) In vitro relative recoveries of bicarbonate and carbondioxide measured with the on-line pH meter at 38°C at various flow rates, as previously described [9] (probe CMA/10, membrane length 3 mm, tube length 30 cm). (b) Influence of the length of the tubing between the probe exit and the on-line pH meter on in vitro recovery of carbondioxide (flow rate 2 µl/min)

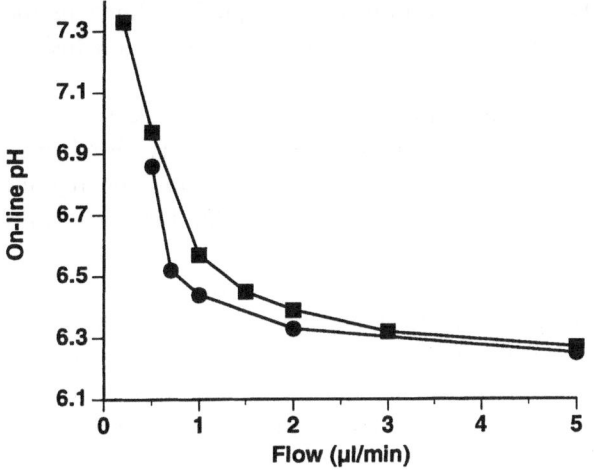

Fig. 2. On-line pH of dialysates from the parietal cortex of two rats, measured at various flow rates (probe CMA/10, membrane length 3 mm, perfusion medium 0.9% NaCl, tube length 30 cm.) The lower the flow rate, the more bicarbonate (higher recovery) and the less CO_2 (more loss through the tubing wall) will remain in the dialysate. At 0.5 µl/min. the pH approaches the value known from the literature [17]

b) Results of the in vivo experiments are shown in Fig. 2. As flow rate was reduced, pH rose and at 0.5 µl/min it approached 7.3, the value reported for extracellular pH by Siesjö et al. [17].

c) Figure 3 shows the measured concentrations of GSH in the dialysates and the corresponding calculated relative recoveries for the given range of outer concentrations. It can be seen that the dialysate concentration is not linearly dependent on the outer concentration; thus relative recovery (%) varies with the outer concentration. Similar results were obtained for Cys.

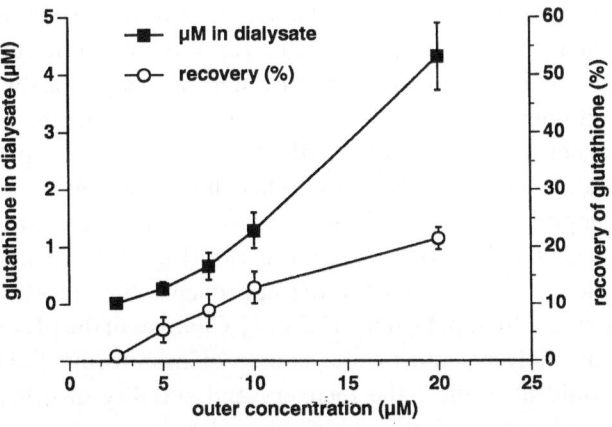

Fig. 3. Concentrations of glutathione in the dialysate, and the calculated corresponding in vitro relative recoveries (both means ± sem, n = 5) at various concentrations of glutathione in the outer medium (probe CMA10, membrane length 3 mm, perfused with Ringer solution

d) The bacterial tests showed one contaminated probe and two negative results. The contamination occurred because of a loose connector between tubing and probe, and was not related to the probe itself. Therefore we assumed that the probes were still undamaged and patent after sterilization with ethylene dioxide at 60 °C.

Measurements in Patients

Parameters which we had detected in rat brain [11] could also be measured in the cortex of patient 1. The results for Asc, UA and GSH are shown in Fig. 4. Values for Cys were: 0.182 µM at 0.5 h; 0.065 µM at 1h; < 0.005 µM at 2h. Baseline levels were already reached after 1 hour. Levels of Asc and GSH, compounds occurring mainly intracellularly, were higher in the first sample after probe insertion, as also found for other parameters in rat models [5].

Results for patient 2 (with a severe head injury) are shown in Table 1. The basal levels obtained by linear

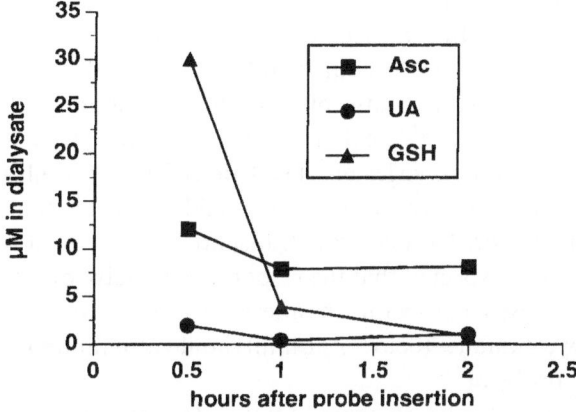

Fig. 4. Basal levels of ascorbic acid, uric acid and glutathione measured during an extra-intracranial bypass operation (probe CMA/12, membrane length 4 mm; perfusion medium, 0.9% saline; flow rate, 2 µl/min)

Table 1. *Effects of a Change in Flow Rate on Levels of Parameters in Cortical Dialysates from a Patient with Head Injury.* The values at zero flow were estimated by linear extrapolation

Flow rate µl/min	Ascorbic acid (µM)	Uric acid (µM)	Cysteine (µM)	Glutathione (µM)
2.0	5.21	1.39	12.84	0.27
1.0	7.82	3.00	18.56	0.45
Estimated zero flow	10.43	4.61	24.28	0.63

extrapolation of values obtained at 2 µl/min and 1 µl/min to virtual no-flow are given in the bottom row. The values for Cys are markedly higher than those found during the bypass operation.

Discussion

Cerebral microdialysis has been thoroughly investigated in multiple animal models (for examples, see [1]. However, before it can be introduced into the clinic as an improved method of cerebral monitoring, certain ethical, methodological and clinical factors must be considered.

Ethical

There are two main critisms of the MD method: first, that there might be damage to the brain tissue caused by the probe, and second, that brain function might be disturbed because substances diffusing into the probe become depleted around the membrane. In fact, we found the volume of irreversibly lesioned tissue around a probe of 4 mm membrane length and 0.5 mm diameter to be about 0.75 to 1.5 mm^3 (unpublished result, see also [2]). In contrast, the catchment volume around the probe measures about 75 to 100 mm^3 (see also [3]). Therefore, with a ratio of 1:100 between lesion and catchment volume we do not expect that "the probe is monitoring its own lesion". Depletion of the extracellular space, e.g. from calcium[1] could affect function, and therefore basal levels of transmitters; however, it is not to be expected that the response to massive events such as ischaemia would be altered. The use of very low flow techniques (below 2 µl/min) should also minimize this problem.

In fact, the lesion caused by the MD probe is minimal compared with the lesion caused by an intracerebral or intraventricular ICP monitoring device. If the clinical picture indicates that cerebral pressure should be monitored, or that a craniotomy is necessary, it is ethically tenable to use an MD probe in the patient. Additionally, in contrast to ICP monitors, which provide information about only one parameter, MD is potentially able to tell us about multiple aspects of brain metabolism.

Depending on the clinical state of the patient in critical care, we want to monitor either pathological tissue to assess the severity of the damage and follow the effects of therapy, or still intact brain tissue to prevent additional damage caused by new secondary lesions. In contrast to most conventional methods, MD enables monitoring of a small volume in the region of special interest. However, direct conclusions about the rest of the brain cannot be drawn in the same way as with ICP or jugular bulb measurement; on the other hand there is less possibility for falsification of the results due to information from regions outside the brain, as is the case for jugular venous blood [16].

Before using an MD probe in humans, we wanted to be sure that there would be no danger of infection through the perfused sterilized probe, although the perfusion medium used (0.9% saline) is also sterile. The results of our bacterial tests showed that this danger is minimal.

We can therefore conclude that ethically there are enough reasons to legitimate the clinical use of MD, provided tactics and logistics are carefully planned.

Methodological

The parameters used must reflect pathological changes in good time, so that the clinician can react with a suitable therapy. Ideally, they should also show specific changes in specific pathological situations. Our experimental results show that it is very important to thoroughly investigate the behaviour of these chosen parameters in the laboratory and in animal models, before applying the parameters in the clinic. For instance, we found that on-line pH values depended on certain factors in the set-up such as tube length and flow. The difference in relative recovery between CO_2 and bicarbonate at different flow rates led to different acid-base balance in the dialysate at each point (Fig. 1a). Another important finding was the dependence of the recovery of CO_2 on the length of tubing between the probe and the pH cell (Fig. 1b). We explain this by the increased loss of CO_2 through the gas-permeable tubing at low flows. Thus it must be realised that inter-experimental or inter-patient comparisons of pH values can only be made when flow rate and tube length are identical. The in vitro findings were confirmed by in vivo experiments in rats (Fig. 2). The lower the flow, the nearer the pH approaches the reported extracellular pH value of 7.3 [17]. Changes of the pH of the dialysate during the course of monitoring [12] could also affect the recovery and stability of other substances, a factor which should be seriously considered.

The in vitro relative recovery of GSH in the expected biological range (Fig. 2) demonstrated for the first time the possibility of a non-linear recovery. Percentage recovery was much lower at low concentrations. This leads to exaggeration of small concentration differences, enhancing the effectivity of monitoring. Factors which may play a role include a threshold behaviour of membrane permeability at low concentrations, and oxidation during sample collection. However, in vivo recovery is quite different from in vitro recovery. It depends on a variety of factors such as tortuosity, as well as uptake, supply and metabolism of the compound of interest in the brain (see e.g. Boutelle and Fillenz, in this volume). There may also be artefacts influencing the results; for instance when an MD probe is used together with an ICP device, there must be enough distance between them to avoid interference with the MD monitoring. All these factors indicate that great care must be taken in the interpretation of MD findings in the clinic, which can only reflect conditions in the ECF to a limited extent.

Clinical

At least one parameter for use in the clinic should be measured on-line, and should react sensitively to metabolic deterioration at an early stage by showing pathological values. The deterioration can then later be confirmed by analysis of other parameters in the fractioned samples. For use in the clinic, the analyses of the samples should be available within a reasonable time. This concept implies that we know the range of "normal" values in minimally damaged brain. A start has been made [6, 13], but values for many parameters will have to be estimated from animal experiments until human values are established. Our first measurements during an extra-intracranial bypass operation from basically healthy cortex allowed us to compare experimental and clinical values of radical scavengers and UA (Fig. 4). In this patient we found values of the same order as those in the rat [11]. Stable values were already reached after 1 hour. The first measurement in a highly pathological cortex, after evacuation of a subdural hematoma with subsequent uncontrollable brain swelling, revealed values for Cys very much higher than those found in basically healthy cortex (Table 1). This might partially be explained by the non-linear recovery described above. Such high levels were also found during focal ischaemia in the rat [11]. However, Asc, UA and GSH, which are also elevated during ischaemia, showed no marked increases. It is evident that much more data will have to be collected before we are able to correlate MD findings with the clinical picture.

Initially, microdialytic monitoring will rarely have a direct impact on therapeutic steps, it will more likely only help to confirm standard clinical practice. This can reduce the original enthusiasm. The so-called "vial business" can have a similar effect; by this we mean the huge number of fractioned dialysate samples which must be analysed in time for clinical consideration. Another important aspect is keeping track of the mutual chronology of parameter changes and clinical events. For this, a modern data collection system would be advantageous. We can conclude that future developments should aim towards on-line analysis of the parameters, similar to our measurement of pH of the dialysate.

Future Aspects

Measurements with different and lower flows (see e.g. Table 1) allow estimation of "true" extracellular values by means of extrapolation to virtual no-flow [8]. A standardised method of very low flow (0.1–0.5 µl/min.) together with a longer membrane, could routinely give a recovery of about 100%, and substance depletion in the tissue would be reduced. Dialysate values would approach the extracellular ones, which would enable inter-patient and inter-clinic comparisons. This method must be combined with improved analytical methods, which are capable of detecting small amounts of substances in volumes of under 10 µl. Otherwise the delay before analysis is too long, and there is danger of substance decay. Additional measures could include very short tubing and cooling of the dialysate. Beside monitoring to prevent secondary lesions, future applications of MD in the clinic could include assessing conventional therapies, confirming hypotheses about pathological mechanisms, or establishing new therapies. Feed-back from MD is more rapid than with conventional means, e.g. assessment of outcome. In the case of unexpected, or even controversial results the clinician should have access to scientific consultation and be able to cooperate in experimental or methodological work. This will be the best way to assess credibility and reproducibility, and to explore the mechanisms which lead to pathological situations in the brain.

To conclude, our hopes for the future are the following: The combination of microdialysis with other methods such as tissue O_2, CO_2 and pH measurements [18], regional cerebral blood flow in the vicinity of the probe (Zauner, this volume) and jugular bulb oxygen saturation (Goodman, this volume) will provide more precise information and enable us to find suitable parameters; standardised apparatus and methods of MD will allow for comparison between patients, and for exchange of data between clinics; development of different membrane types could also give the chance to measure other larger neurochemical substances of clinical interest.

References

1. Benveniste H (1989) Brain microdialysis. J Neurochem 52: 1667–1679
2. Benveniste H, Diemer NH (1987) Cellular reactions to implantation of a microdialysis tube in the rat hippocampus. Acta Neuropathol (Berl) 74: 234–238
3. Benveniste H, Huttemeier PC (1990) Microdialysis—theory and application. Prog Neurobiol 35: 195–215
4. Graham DI, Ford I, Adams JH, Doyle D, Teasdale GM, Lawrence AE, McLellan DR (1989) Ischaemic brain damage is still common in fatal non-missile head injury. J Neurol Neurosurg Psychiatry 52: 346–350
5. Hillered L, Hallstrom A, Segersvard S, Persson L, Ungerstedt U (1989) Dynamics of extracellular metabolites in the striatum after middle cerebral artery occlusion in the rat monitored by intracerebral microdialysis, (published erratum appears in J Cereb Blood Flow Metab 10(1): 149–151, 1990). J Cereb Blood Flow Metab 9: 607–616
6. Hillered L, Persson L, Ponten U, Ungerstedt U (1990) Neurometabolic monitoring of the ischaemic human brain using microdialysis. Acta Neurochir (Wien) 102: 91–97
7. Honegger, CG, Langemann H, Krenger W, Kempf A (1989) Liquid chromatographic determination of common water-soluble antioxidants in biological samples. J Chromatogr 487: 463–468
8. Jacobson J, Sandberg M, Hamberger A (1985) Mass transfer in brain dialysis devices—a new method for the estimation of extracellular amino acids. J Neurosci Meth 15: 263–268
9. Landolt H, Langemann H, Gratzl O (1993) On-line monitoring of cerebral pH by microdialysis. Neurosurgery 32: 1000–1004
10. Landolt H, Langemann H, Mendelowitsch A, Gratzl O (1994) Neurochemical monitoring and on-line pH measurements using brain microdialysis in patients in intensive care. Acta Neurochir (Wien) [Suppl] 60: 475–478
11. Landolt H, Lutz TW, Langemann H, Stauble D, Mendelowitsch A, Gratzl O, Honegger CG (1992) Extracellular antioxidants and amino acids in the cortex of the rat—monitoring by microdialysis of early ischaemic changes. J Cereb Blood Flow Metab 12: 96–102
12. Langemann H, Mendelowitsch A, Landolt H, Alessandri B, Gratzl O (1995) Experimental and clinical monitoring of glucose by microdialysis. Clin Neurol Neurosurg 97: 149–155
13. Mendelowitsch A, Langemann H, Landolt H, Gratzl O (1994) Microdialytic monitoring of ischemic changes during brain retraction for aneursym surgery. In: Nagai H, Kamiya K *et al* (eds) Ninth International Symposium on Intercranial Pressure. Springer, Berlin Heidelberg New York Tokyo, pp 260–263
14. Mindermann T, Landolt H, Zimmerli W, Rajacic Z, Gratzl O (1993) Penetration of rifampicin into the brain tissue and cerebral extracellular space of rats. J Antimicrob Chemother 31: 731–737
15. Persson L, Hillered L (1992) Chemical monitoring of neurosurgical intensive care patients using intracerebral microdialysis. J Neurosurg 76: 72–80
16. Robertson C, Narayan R, Gokoslan Z, Pahwa R, Grossman R, Caram P, Allen E (1989) Cerebral arteriovenous difference as an estimate of cerebral blood flow in comatose patients. J Neurosurg 70: 222–230
17. Siesjö B, von Hanwehr R, Nergellius G, Nevander G, Ingvar M (1985) Extra- and intracellular pH in the brain during seizures and in the recovery period following the arrest of seizure activity. J Cereb Blood Flow Metab 5: 47–57
18. Zauner A, Bullock R, Young H (1985) Brain oxygen, CO_2 and cerebral blood flow measurements in focal ischaemia. J Cereb Blood Flow Metab 15: S297

Correspondence: H. Landolt, M.D., Neurosurgical Clinic, Kantonsspital, CH-5000 Aarau, Switzerland.

Acta Neurochir (1996) [Suppl] 67: 37–39

Lactic Acid and Amino Acid Fluctuations Measured Using Microdialysis Reflect Physiological Derangements in Head Injury

J.C. Goodman, S.P. Gopinath, A.B. Valadka, R.K. Narayan, R.G. Grossman, R.K. Simpson Jr., and **C.S. Robertson**

Departments of Neurosurgery and Pathology, Baylor College of Medicine, Houston, TX, U.S.A.

Summary

We examined the extracellular neurochemical milieu in 34 head injured patients using microdialysis while simultaneously monitoring intracranial pressure, cerebral perfusion pressure, and jugular venous oxygen saturation. Derangements of anaerobic metabolism reflected by increased lactate and lactate/pyruvate ratios, and release of amino acids were seen at the same time as physiological deterioration in the majority of instances. Clinical microdialysis may provide insights into the neurochemistry of head injury, and such information may lead to new methods of monitoring and treating head injured patients.

Keywords: Head injury; microdialysis; lactic acid; amino acids; glutamate aspartate; excitotoxicity; ischemia.

Introduction

Lactic acidosis and release of excitotoxic amino acids are important neurochemical signatures of secondary brain damage following head injury [1–6]. Microdialysis is a promising method to permit monitoring of these neurochemical alterations in the intensive care setting [7–17]. We studied the chemical composition of extracellular space of the brain continuously sampled using microdialysis in 34 brain injured patients, and correlated these neurochemical data with intracranial pressure, jugular venous oxygen saturation, and clinical events including barbiturate coma and brain death.

Materials and Methods

The 34 patients were predominantly young men reflecting the epidemiology of head trauma in the United States. Their injuries included cerebral contusion (n=15), epidural hematoma (n=4), subdural hematoma (n=21), intracerebral hematoma (n=4), and penetrating gunshot wound (n=2). Some individuals had multiple types of injury.

Microdialysis probes were placed via burrhole or craniotomy in the cerebral cortex. Probes were placed at the time of intracranial pressure monitor placement or at craniotomy for decompression of hematoma or contusion. The cerebral cortex was directly visualized and the probes were placed in grossly normal appearing cortex. The 5 mm loop microdialysis probes were constructed using 30,000 molecular weight cutoff dialysis tubing. The loop was inserted obliquely into the cerebral cortex and the probe was lightly secured to the dura allowing some slack in the infusion and collection lines permitting the probe to move with the brain rather than extending rigidly into the cortical parenchyma potentially damaging the cortex. The probe was confined to the cerebral cortex with no sampling of subcortical structures. The delicate inflow and outflow lines of the probe ran through a length of plastic tubing serving as a protective umbilical cord leading to the microfraction collector and pump at the bedside (CMA/Microdialysis AB, Stockholm, Sweden).

Medical grade 0.9% intravenous infusion saline solution was used as the dialysate. While artificial CSF would theoretically be a more suitable dialysate, physiological saline is readily available, sterile, pyrogen-free, calcium-free, and devoid of lactic acid and amino acids. Dialysate was collected in 30 minute epochs using a refrigerated bedside fraction collector. The dialysate flow rate was 2 μl/minute and analyte recovery was 9 to 11% during in vitro probe calibration against lactate and amino acids.

Organic and amino acid analyses were performed using high pressure liquid chromatography (HPLC) [15, 18–23]. Lactate and pyruvate measurements were performed by HPLC using a 25 μl injection of unprocessed microdialysate onto a BioRad HP × 87 anion exchange organic acid column perfused isocratically with dilute sulfuric acid (BioRad Laboratories, Hercules, Ca). Amino acid analysis was performed using pre-column phenylisocyanate (PITC) derivatization with subsequent gradient programed reverse phase chromatography with UV absorbance detection (Waters Associates, PICO-TAG, Milford, MA).

Increased analyte levels could reflect neurochemical derangements in the brain, but they may also have resulted from impaired dialysate flow with subsequent increased analyte recovery. We guarded against this possibility by pre-weighing and labelling the fraction collection vials, and then weighting the vials after the samples were collected. The sample volume of 60 microliters expected in an unimpeded collection epoch raised the weight of the vial by 60 mg. We found that there was sufficient variability in vial weights that pre-weighing was an essential though tedious requirement rather than simply weighing the vials once after collection of the samples. If the sample volumes were lower than 60 microliters, then the vial was rejected for analysis and the third vial after resumption of normal sample volumes was used. Lactate analyses have been completed in 32/34 patients and amino acid analyses have been completed in 23/34. Neurochemical analyses were performed without knowledge of physiological monitoring data.

A total of 1534 hours of microdialysis monitoring was performed. Continuous intracranial pressure (ICP), mean arterial pressure (MAP), cerebral perfusion pressure (CPP), and jugular venous oxygen saturation (SjvO$_2$) measurements were obtained concurrently with microdialysis monitoring. For tabulating our results, we defined a pathophysiological event to be ICP > 25 mmHg unresponsive to therapy or SjvO$_2$ < 50% for 10 minutes or more. In some cases, local cerebral blood flow (CBF) was measured using a cortical surface thermodilution probe. Additionally, two instances of barbiturate coma and one case of brain death were examined. The microdialysis sample collection times were linked to the physiological data stream permitting graphic display of the information using a commercially available relational database (Paradox for Windows, Borland, Scotts Valley, CA). This display facilitates visual correlation of multiple physiological and neurochemical events.

Results

Pathophysiological events occurred in 53% of patients during neurochemical monitoring. Elevations of lactate and lactate/pyruvate ratios were seen during episodes of jugular venous oxygen desaturation, increased intracranial pressure, and in brain death. Decreased lactate and lactate/pyruvate ratios were seen when barbiturate coma was instituted, but in one instance the barbiturate coma eventually failed to control increased intracranial pressure and this failure was accompanied by a progressive elevation of microdialysate lactate. A total of 27 lactate elevations were seen, and 21/27 (78%) of these were accompanied by a pathophysiological event. A total of 24 pathophysiological events were detected, and 21/24 (87.5%) were associated with elevations of lactate.

The excitatory amino acids glutamate and aspartate, the inhibitory amino acid and NMDA receptor obligate co-agonist glycine, and the putative glial osmoregulatory amino acid taurine were also elevated during jugular venous oxygen desaturation, intractable increased intracranial pressure, and in brain death. In most instances, the excitatory amino acids increased in concert with lactate and corresponded to a physiologically identifiable jugular venous oxygen desaturation or intracranial pressure elevation. The excitatory amino acids in the extracellular space decreased with the institution of barbiturate coma. In the case of brain death, all amino acids rose, attaining levels in the hundreds of micromoles indicating widespread cellular breakdown. Local cerebral blood flow measured by thermodilution in this patient was negligible.

No infectious complications resulted from microdialysis monitoring. In one case (1/34, 3%), a small intraparenchymal hematoma developed near the microdialysis probe site. The hematoma was also near a pressure transducer which was substantially larger than the microdialysis probe.

Discussion

Elevations of lactate and the lactate/pyruvate ratio correlate with pathophysiological events. These neurochemical indicators of anaerobic tissue metabolism corroborate the significant role of ischemic injury as a mechanism of secondary injury in head trauma as has been suggested by pathological, cerebral blood flow, jugular venous oxygen saturation, and PET scan studies.

Our study also shows that elevations of the excitatory amino acids glutamate and aspartate occur during pathophysiological events. These findings support the role of excitotoxicity in secondary brain injury. Additionally, the inhibitory amino acid glycine is elevated, and this amino acid also may play a role in excitotoxicity as it is an obligatory co-agonist of the NMDA receptor [1, 2, 5, 6, 24–26]. The elevation of taurine was intriguing because this amino acid is thought to have a role in astrocyte osmoregulation, and its elevation may reflect deranged glial volume regulation following head injury [27]. The extraordinary elevations of all amino acids in brain death are not unexpected, but serve to emphasize the potential toxic effect of areas of brain necrosis on adjacent viable brain tissue due to the release of excitoxins.

This study demonstrates that neurochemical monitoring using microdialysis is feasible in neurosurgical patients, and can provide insights into the biochemical events after brain injury. Correlation was obtained between worsening neurological state and elevations of lactic acid and amino acids. If threshold concentrations of these analytes corresponding to tissue damage or poor clinical outcome can be established, it may be desirable to develop rapid analysis systems capable of giving intensive care physicians immediate information about neurochemical deterioration in their head injured patients.

Acknowledgements

The authors gratefully acknowledge the excellent support of the nursing staff and neurosurgical house officers of the Neurosurgical Intensive Care Unit, Ben Taub General Hospital, Houston, Texas, and the technical staff of the Neurochemical Research Laboratory, Department of Neurosurgery, Baylor College of Medicine. This work was supported by NIH PO1-NS27616.

References

1. Siesjo BK (1992) Pathophysiology and treatment of focal cerebral ischemia—part I: pathophysiology. J Neurosurg 77: 169–184

2. Siesjo B (1992) Pathophysiology and treatment of focal cerebral ischemia—part II: mechanisms of damage and treatment. J Neurosurg 77: 337–354

3. Pitts LH, McIntosh TK (1990) Dynamic changes after brain trauma. In: Braakman R (ed) Head injury. Revised series, 13 Ed. Elsevier, New York, pp 65–100 (Vinken PJ, Bruyn GW, Klawans HL (ed) Handbook of clinical neurology, Vol 57)

4. Hovda DA, Becker DP, Katayama Y (1992) Secondary injury and acidosis. J Neurotrauma 9 [Suppl 1]: 47–60

5. Globus MYT, Dietrich WD (1992) The role of neurotransmitters in brain injury. 1st Ed. Plenum, New York: p 378.

6. Benveniste H (1991) The excitotoxin hypothesis in relation to cerebral ischemia. Cerebrovasc Brain Metab Rev 3(3): 213–245

7. Hamberger A, Jacobson I, Nystrom B, Sandberg M (1991) Microdialysis sampling of the neuronal environment in basic and clinical research. J Intern Med 230(4): 375–380

8. Hillered L, Persson L, Ponten U, Ungerstedt U (1990) Neurometabolic monitoring of the ischaemic human brain using microdialysis. Acta Neurochir (Wien) 102(3–4): 91–97

9. Hillered L, Persson L (1991) Microdialysis for metabolic monitoring in cerebral ischemia and trauma: experimental and clinical studies. In: Robinson TE, Justice Jr JB (eds) Microdialysis in the neurosciences, 1st Ed. Elsevier, New York, p 450 (Huston JP (ed) Techniques in the behavioral and neural sciences, Vol 7)

10. Hillered L, Kotwica Z, Ungerstedt U (1991) Interstitial and cerebrospinal fluid levels of energy-related metabolites after middle cerebral artery occlusion in rats. Exp Med 191: 219–225

11. Lonnroth P (1991) Microdialysis—a new and promising method in clinical medicine. J Intern Med 230: 363–364

12. Meyerson BA, Linderoth B, Karlsson H, Ungerstedt U (1990) Microdialysis in the human brain: extracellular measurements in the thalamus of parkinsonian patients. Life Sci 46(4): 301–308

13. Persson L, Hillered L (1992) Chemical monitoring of neurosurgical intensive care patients using intracerebral microdialysis. J Neurosurg 76(1): 72–80

14. Robinson TE, Justice Jr JB (1991) Microdialysis in the neurosciences, 1st ed. Elsevier, New York, p 450 (Huston JP (ed) Techniques in the behavioral and neural sciences, Vol 7)

15. Ronne EE, Hillered L, Flink R, Spannare B, Ungerstedt U, Carlson H (1992) Intracerebral microdialysis of extracellular amino acids in the human epileptic focus. J Cereb Blood Flow Metab 12(5): 873–876

16. Ungerstedt U (1991) Microdialysis—principles and applications for studies in animals and man. J Intern Med 230: 365–373

17. Whittle IR (1990) Intracerebral microdialysis: a new method in applied clinical neuroscience research editorial. Br J Neurosurg 4(6): 459–462

18. Eklund T, Wahlberg J, Ungerstedt U, Hillered L (1991) Interstitial lactate, inosine and hypoxanthine in rat kidney during normothermic ischaemia and recirculation. Acta Physiol Scand 143(3): 279–286

19. Hallstrom A, Carlsson A, Hillered L, Ungerstedt U (1989) Simultaneous determination of lactate, pyruvate, and ascorbate in microdialysis samples from rat brain, blood, fat, and muscle using high-performance liquid chromatography. J Pharmacol Methods 22(2): 113–124

20. Inao S, Marmarou A, Clarke GD, Andersen BJ, Fatouros PP, Young HF (1988) Production and clearance of lactate from brain tissue, cerebrospinal fluid, and serum following experimental brain injury. J Neurosurg 69: 736–744

21. Nilsson P, Hillered L, Ponten U, Ungerstedt U (1990) Changes in cortical extracellular levels of energy-related metabolites and amino acids following concussive brain injury in rats. J Cereb Blood Flow Metab 19: 631–637

22. Robertson CS, Goodman JC, Grossman RG, Priessman A (1990) Reduction in spinal cord post-ischemic lactic acidosis and functional improvement with dichloroacetate. J Neurotrauma 7: 1–12

23. Simpson RK, Robertson CS, Goodman JC (1990) Spinal cord ischemia-induced elevation of amino acids: extracellular measurement with microdialysis. Neurochem Res 15(6): 635–639

24. Rothman SM, Olney JW (1986) Glutamate and the pathophysiology of hypoxic-ischemic brain damage. Ann Neurol 19: 105–111

25. Palmer AM, Marion DW, Botscheller ML, Swedlow PE, Styren SD, DeKosky ST (1993) Traumatic brain injury-induced excitotoxicity assessed in a controlled cortical impact model. J Neurochem 61: 2015–2024

26. Tsumoto T (1990) Excitatory amino acid transmitters and their receptors in neural circuits of the cerebral neocortex. Neurosci Res 9: 79–102

27. Schousboe A, Pasantes-Morales H (1992) Role of taurine in neural cell volume regulation. Can J Physiol Pharmacol 70 [Suppl]: 356–361

Correspondence: J. Clay Goodman, M.D., Department of Pathology, Baylor College of Medicine, One Baylor Plaza, Houston, TX 77030, U.S.A.

Acta Neurochir (1996) [Suppl] 67: 40–44

Glutamate Release and Cerebral Blood Flow After Severe Human Head Injury

A. Zauner, R. Bullock, A.J. Kuta, J. Woodward, and H.F. Young

Division of Neurosurgery, Medical College of Virginia, Virginia Commonwealth University, Richmond, VA, U.S.A.

Summary

Elevations of extracellular glutamate have been found in patients with prolonged brain ischemia and focal cerebral contusions, following severe head injury. About 30% of severely head injured patients develop cerebral ischemia, defined as CBF < 18 ml/100g/min. Patients with both global and regional cerebral ischemia have the worst outcome. However, the relationship between CBF and EAA release is not well understood in head injured humans, and may differ from the findings in normal animals. To study the relationship between EAA release and CBF after severe head injury, we performed cerebral blood flow measurements using stable xenon enhanced computed tomography and correlated these with glutamate release in the extracellular fluid, measured by continuous microdialysis, in 25 severely head injured patients.

Sustained cerebral blood flow reductions below the threshold for ischemic neuronal damage was closely related to massive excitatory amino acid release, as in previous animal studies. In patients without secondary ischemia, or focal contusions, delayed post-traumatic glutamate release appeared to be only transient or did not occur at all.

Keywords: Extracellular glutamate release; cerebral blood flow; brain ischemia; severe head injury.

Introduction

Many animal models have demonstrated striking accumulation of excitatory aminoacids (EAA's) during brain ischemia, using microdialysis [1, 13, 23]. The most important EAA neurotransmitter is glutamate, because of its neurotoxicity, and it has now become a major focus for development of selective pharmacological antagonists as neuroprotectants [3, 4, 21]. Calciummediated damage to intracellular structures and the generation of free radicals are important biochemical consequences following shearing injury and ischemic damage. The release of large concentrations of extracellular EAA's appears to account for the majority of this calcium influx in pathological situations [3, 5, 21]. Experimental studies have demonstrated up to a sevenfold extracellular fluid (ECF) glutamate in-

crease in models of shearing injury and subdural hematoma, and up to a 40-fold increase after focal ischemia [8, 11, 18]. Shimada *et al.*, in a global model of brain ischemia, have demonstrated a 30-fold increase in glutamate, when the CBF fell below a blood flow threshold of 20 ml/100g/min [22]. In the same study, the non-neurotransmitter aminoacids (taurine, alanine, serine, glutamine) increased only slightly, and essential aminoacids (phenylalanine, valine, leucine) did not change at all during global ischemia, suggesting that presynaptic vesicular glutamate release was responsible. These large increases in ECF excitatory amino acid neurotransmitters below a blood flow threshold sufficient to induce functional disturbance, supports the role of these amino acids in the causation of ischemic cell damage. However, the relationship between EAA release and CBF after trauma may be profoundly different from that which is seen in ischemia. Moderate traumatic injury has been shown to render the brain significantly more vulnerable to secondary ischemic damage, in animal models, and this may be ameliorated by pretreatment with glutamate antagonists [9, 12, 15].

The aim of our current human study was therefore to test the hypothesis that CBF, in severely head injured patients, is a major determinant of glutamate release.

Patients and Methods

This study was approved by the Committee on the Conduct of Human Research at the Medical College of Virginia, Virginia Commonwealth University.

Microdialysis

A 10 mm flexible microdialysis probe with an external diameter of 0.5 mm was used. The probe was inserted into cortex, either at craniotomy, or via a ventriculostomy twist drill site. Care was taken

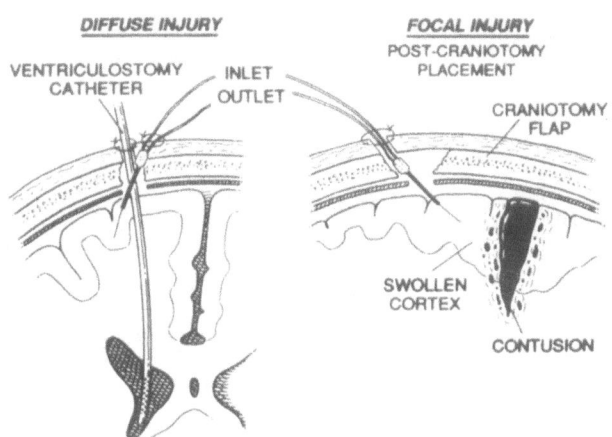

Fig. 1. Microdialysis in human head injury. Placement of micro-dialysis probe at the site of ventriculostomy, or during surgery, next to a cerebral contusion. The tip of the probe is directed away from the ventricular catheter

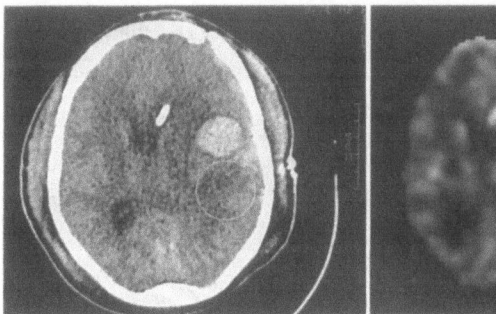
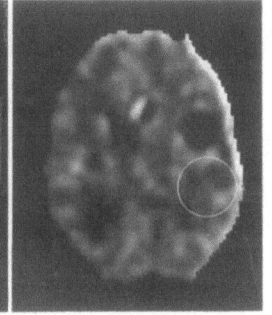

Fig. 2. Baseline CT scan and corresponding CBF image with region of interest, next to a contusion where the microdialysis probe was placed (the microdialysis probe is not radiodense)

that the tip of the microdialysis probe was pointed away from the ventricular catheter (Fig. 1). Intraoperatively, the probe was placed into damaged, but viable tissue after decompression and/or clot removal. Thereafter in the intensive care unit, the probe was perfused at 2 microliters per minute using sterile 0.9% saline. 60 μl dialysates were collected every 30 minutes, into sealed glass tubes using a refrigerated (4°C) automated collector system (CMA 170 system, CMA/Microdialysis, Acton, MA). The microdialysis probe was left in place for up to 4 days and saved thereafter for in vitro calibration. Glutamate was measured using high performance liquid chromatography (HPLC). Clinical events and the dialysate sampling times were logged into a mainframe computer, together with arterial blood pressure, intracranial pressure and $ETCO_2$.

Cerebral Blood Flow (CBF) Measurements

We used stable (non-radioactive) xenon-enhanced computed tomography for measuring cerebral blood flow [2, 19, 24]. This is performed by repeated CT scanning during the inhalation of a gas mixture containing 30% xenon, 40% oxygen and room air. This method computes blood flow in ml/100g/min, by measuring the brain tissue uptake during arterial build-up of the xenon concentration, which is converted into Houndsfield units [10, 17]. At the beginning of each study, two baseline, non-enhanced scans were obtained at three brain levels determined by the diagnostic CT scan. Eight sequential CT scans at each level were obtained during an 8 minutes wash-out study [2].

End-tidal xenon, blood pressure, heart rate, end-tidal $PaCO_2$, O_2 saturation and intracranial pressure (follow-up studies only) were monitored throughout each study.

The CBF studies were done on admission (except in patients who underwent emergency surgery or were hemodynamically unstable), and on day 4 ± 1. CBF images were analyzed, using a 20–30 mm² region of interest (ROI), around the site where the microdialysis probe was placed (Fig. 2). Hemispheric blood flow was also calculated by outlining the hemisphere, using drawing tools on the CT screen.

Statistical Analysis

For each patient, both the mean glutamate release for the 3 to 6 hour period closest to the time of CBF measurement, as well as the peak glutamate values were calculated, and compared to CBF measurements (regional CBF = ROI, and hemispheric CBF). Descriptive statistics, regression analysis, and nonparametric tests were used for analysis.

Results

In 25 severely head injured patients, GCS $\leqslant 8$, extracellular glutamate release was monitored for periods from 20 hours to 4 days (4 patients died within 48 hours of injury). In vitro calibration of the probes, revealed a recovery rate for EAA's of $43 \pm 5\%$. 7 patients had emergency surgery and a total of 42 CBF measurements between 1 hour and 5 days after injury were done. Not all patients received two CBF studies, because some underwent emergency surgery on admission, and some died prior to the second study, on day 4 ± 1. In some patients, glutamate was markedly increased for several hours only, and often this could not be related to clinical events such as sustained increases in ICP (despite therapy) or documented hypoperfusion. The mean glutamate release and CBF values of a patient with a good outcome and a patient who died after secondary ischemic events are shown in Figs. 3 and 4, respectively.

Glutamate Release and Regional CBF

There was a significant correlation between mean glutamate release (over 3–6 hours) and the regional cerebral blood flow measurements (Spearman Rank Correlation, $p < 0.001$, regression analysis, $R^2 = 0.895$), Fig. 5. There was no relationship between peak glutamate release for each patient, and regional CBF ($R^2 = 0.299$). All patients with a regional CBF of less than 16 ml/100g/min had a mean regional dialysate glutamate value of more than 20 μMol/l. CBF measurements between 16 and 28 ml/100g/min had

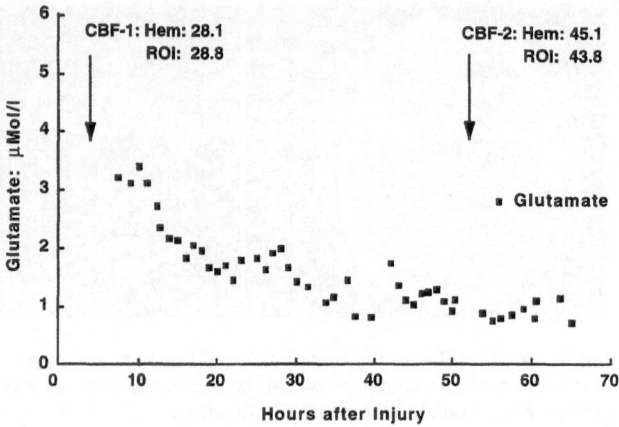

Fig. 3. Patient 1. Severely head injured patient (initial GCS = 6, diffuse brain injury), who recovered completely from injury. The initial CBF study was done 3 hours after injury, and was 28 ml/100 g/min for hemispheric (*Hem*) and regional (*ROI*) blood flow. Glutamate release was slightly increased for the first 12 hours after injury but returned to baseline values. Normal CBF on day 3 after injury

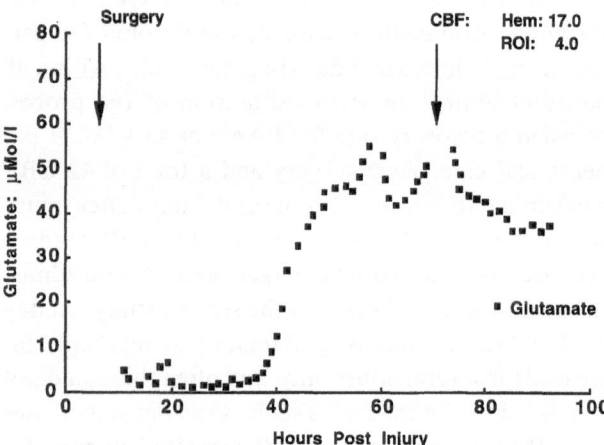

Fig. 4. Patient 2. Severely head injured patient (initial GCS = 3, acute subdural hematoma), who died on day 5. Emergency surgery was performed on admission, without an initial CBF study. Massive increase of glutamate seen after 50 hours post injury. A CBF study on day 4 showed very low regional flow (*ROI*), and hemispheric blood flow (*Hem*), at the ischemic threshold (17 ml/100 g/min)

glutamate levels ranging between 5 and 20 μMol/l. All patients with normal CBF or relative hyperemia, had glutamate levels below 5 μMol/l.

Hemispheric CBF

Even though the 10 mm microdialysis probe only measures glutamate in a relatively small brain volume (probably about 4 cm³), the mean glutamate release was closely correlated with hemispheric CBF (p < 0.001,

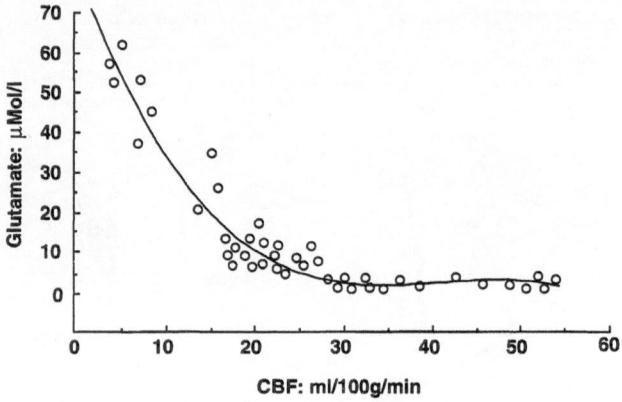

Fig. 5. Relationship between cerebral blood flow measurements, and extracellular glutamate, after severe head injury (n = 25 patients, $R^2 = 0.895$, p < 0.001). Note that a threshold for glutamate release exists, at about 18–20 ml/100 g/min

$R^2 = 0.632$). Hemispheric CBF showed no relationship to peak glutamate levels ($R^2 = 0.198$).

Discussion

Our results demonstrate a close relationship between cerebral blood flow and glutamate release in patients after severe head injury. Sustained CBF below the ischemic threshold of 18 ml/100g/min was associated with massively increased extracellular glutamate.

Jones and coworkers showed loss of cellular function at CBF levels below 23 ml/100g/min, in normal, awake monkeys [16]. Infarction occurred when flow levels of 10 ml/100g/min were maintained for more than 3 hours duration, and after 4 hours at a flow value of 18 ml/100g/min. As long as CBF stayed above 18 ml/100g/min, neurons survived, but (temporarily) lost their function. In a feline model of global brain ischemia, extracellular glutamate rose almost immediately after onset of ischemia (CBF < 10 ml/100g/min) and increased to 30 times normal levels after 2 hours [23]. Even though an infarction threshold of 18 ml/100g/min has been adopted by a number of researchers and clinicians [2, 13, 19, 24] the threshold for ischemia may be different after head injury, and in the normal brain [10, 15, 25].

The release of excitatory aminoacids after brain injury or ischemia, has been intensively studied in animal models, in recent years. This is because it has been shown that cerebral ECF glutamate plays an important role in the pathogenesis of selective neuronal injury, infarction and cell swelling. In accordance with the excitotoxic hypothesis, glutamate, released in high concentrations during ischemia, leads to cell damage and neuronal death. Microdialysis studies played an important role in the development of this hypothesis [1, 6, 14, 20, 21]. Animal models have demonstrated a 5–10 fold increase in glutamate, in the cortex and up to a 40 fold increase in the striatum during ischemia [14, 22, 23]. Shearing injury and subdural hematoma models have demonstrated a sevenfold increase in glutamate after injury [3–5, 8].

We speculate that microdialysis studies will continue to play an important role in the development of the role of the "excitotoxic" process in trauma and ischemia. Clinically, such studies can resolve the "window of opportunity" for glutamate antagonists, and can allow selection of patients likely to benefit from such therapy. In humans, we have shown that the magnitude of excitatory aminoacid release during ischemia is even higher and occurs much longer [6, 7]. In 1992, Persson and Hillered [20] demonstrated that long term monitoring of the extracellular microenvironment was feasible in the intensive care unit. We have modified this technique for continuous use over up to four days, in patients after severe head injury [6, 7]. A total of 43 patients have been studied so far at our institution. The pattern of EAA release was mainly determined by the magnitude and type of the initial injury, along with early events prior to stabilization. Patients with uncomplicated injuries demonstrated only a slight EAA increase for a few hours, or not at all. However, if secondary events, like cerebral hypoperfusion, or a sustained ICP increase (unresponsive to therapy) took place, then a massive EAA release was seen [6]. The persistence of this EAA release for several days, and the greater magnitude of release in humans, may be due to the very much larger volume of ischemically damaged tissue relative to the dialyzing surface of the microdialysis probe in humans, compared to rats. Our current study suggests that a persistent release of glutamate may be involved in delayed brain swelling (penumbral astrocyte swelling, ionic leakage and calcium entry) and occurs simultaneously with CBF levels below the ischemic threshold.

We conclude that sustained cerebral blood flow reductions below the threshold for ischemic neuronal damage (± 18 ml/100g/min) is closely related to massive excitatory amino acid release, as in previous animal studies. In patients without secondary ischemic complications or focal contusions, delayed post-traumatic glutamate release appears to be only transient or does not occur at all. These studies have clear implications for the construction of clinical trials with glutamate antagonists.

References

1. Benveniste H, Drejer J, Schousboe A, Diemer NH (1984) Elevation of the extracellular concentrations of glutamate and aspartate in rat hippocampus during transient cerebral ischemia monitored by intracerebral microdialysis. J Neurochem 43: 1369–1374
2. Bouma GJ, Muizelaar JP, Stringer WA, Choi SC, Fatouros PP, Young HF (1992) Ultra-early evaluation of regional cerebral blood flow in severely head-injured patients using xenon-enhanced computerized tomography. J Neurosurg 77: 360–368
3. Bullock R, Fujisawa H (1992) The role of glutamate antagonists for the treatment of CNS injury. J Neurotrauma 9 [Suppl 2]: S3443–S3461
4. Bullock R (1993) Opportunities for neuroprotective drugs in clinical management of head injury. J Emerg Med 11: 23–30
5. Bullock R (1993) Pathophysiological alterations in the central nervous system due to trauma. Schweiz Med Wochenschr 123: 449–458
6. Bullock R, Zauner A, Tsuji O, Woodward JJ, Young HF, Marmarou AT (1994) Excitatory amino acid release after severe human head trauma: effect of intracranial pressure and cerebral perfusion pressure changes. In: Nagai H et al (eds) Intracranial pressure IX. Springer, Berlin Heidelberg New York Tokyo, pp 264–267
7. Bullock R, Zauner A, Tsuji O, Woodward JJ, Marmarou AT, Young HF (1995) Patterns of excitatory amino acid release and ionic flux after severe head trauma. In: Tsubakawa et al (eds) Neurochemical brain monitoring. Springer, Berlin Heidelberg New York Tokyo, pp 64–71
8. Butcher SP, Bullock R, Graham DL, McCulloch J (1990) Correlation between amino acid release and neuropathological outcome in rat striatum and cortex following middle cerebral artery occlusion. Stroke 21: 1727–1733
9. Chen MH, Bullock R, Graham DL, Miller JD, McCulloch J (1991) Ischemic neuronal damage after acute subdural hematoma in the rat: effects of pretreatment with a glutamate antagonist. J Neurosurg 74: 944–950
10. Drayer BP, Wolfson SK, Reinmuth OM, Dujovny M, Boehnke M, Cook EE (1978) Xenon-enhanced CT for analysis of cerebral integrity, perfusion and blood flow. Stroke 9: 123–130
11. Hayes R, Jenkins LW, Lyeth BG (1992) Neurotransmitter mediated mechanisms of traumatic brain injury: acetylcholine and excitatory amino acids. J Neurotrauma 9 [Suppl 1]: S 173
12. Hayes RL, Jenkins LW, Lyeth BG, Balster RL, Robinson SE, Clifton GL, Stubbins JF, Young HF (1988) Pretreatment with phencyclidine, an N-methyl-D-aspartate antagonist, attenuates long-term behavioral deficits in the rat produced by traumatic brain injury. J Neurotrauma 5: 259–274
13. Heiss WD, Hayakawa T, Waltz AG (1976) Cortical neuronal function during ischemia. Arch Neurol 33: 813–820
14. Hillered L, Hallström A, Segersvärd S, Persson L, Ungerstedt U (1989) Dynamics of extracellular metabolites in the striatum after middle cerebral artery occlusion in the rat monitored by intracerebral microdialysis. J Cereb Blood Flow Metab 9: 607–616
15. Jenkins LW, Moszynski K, Lyeth BG (1989) Increased vulnerability of the mildly traumatized rat brain to cerebral ischemia: the use of controlled secondary ischemia as a research tool to identify common or different mechanisms contributing to mechanical and ischemic brain injury. Brain Res 477: 211–224
16. Jones TH, Morawetz RB, Crowell RM (1981) Thresholds of focal cerebral ischemia in awake monkeys. J Neurosurg 54: 773–782
17. Meyer JS, Hayman LA, Yamamoto M, Sakai F, Nakajima S (1980) Local cerebral blood flow measured by CT after stable xenon inhalation. AJNR 1: 213–215

18. Miller JD, Bullock R, Graham DI, Chen MH, Teadsdale GM (1990) Ischemic brain damage in a model of acute subdural hematoma. Neurosurgery 27: 433–439
19. Muizelaar JP, Schröder ML (1994) Overview of monitoring of cerebral blood flow and metabolism after severe head injury: results and impact on ICU management. Can J Neurol Sci 21: 1–6
20. Persson L, Hillered L (1992) Chemical monitoring of neurosurgical intensive care patients using intracerebral microdialysis. J Neurosurg 76: 72–80
21. Rothman SM, Olney JW (1987) Excitotoxicity and the NMDA receptor. Trends Neurosci 10: 299–302
22. Shimada N, Graf R, Rosner G, Heiss WD (1990) Differences in ischemia-induced accumulation of amino acids in the cat cortex. Stroke 21: 1445–1451
23. Shimada N, Graf R, Rosner G, Heiss WD (1993) Ischemia-induced accumulation of extracellular amino acids in cerebral cortex, white matter, and cerebrospinal fluid. J Neurochem 60: 66–71
24. Schröder ML, Muizelaar JP, Kuta AJ (1994) Documented reversal of global ischemia immediately after removal of an acute subdural hematoma. J Neurosurg 80: 324–327
25. Schröder ML, Muizelaar JP, Kuta AJ, Choi SC (1995) Thresholds for cerebral ischemia after severe head injury: relationship with late CT findings and outcome. J Neurotrauma 13: 17–23

Correspondence: Alois Zauner, M.D., Division of Neurosurgery, Medical College of Virginia, Virginia Commonwealth University, MCV Station, P.O. Box 980 631, Richmond, VA 23298, U.S.A.

Acta Neurochir (1996) [Suppl] 67: 45–47

Increased Levels of Glutamate in Patients with Subarachnoid Haemorrhage as Measured by Intracerebral Microdialysis

O.G. Nilsson, H. Säveland, F. Boris-Möller[1], **L. Brandt,** and **T. Wieloch**[1]

Departments of Neurosurgery and [1]Experimental Brain Research, Lund University Hospital, Lund, Sweden

Summary

Cerebral ischemia associated with subarachnoid haemorrhage (SAH) may have severe consequences for neuronal function leading to reversible or permanent neurological deficits. The excitatory amino acid neurotransmitters, such as glutamate, have been shown to be of particular importance for ischemic neuronal damage. In seven patients who underwent early surgery for a ruptured intracranial aneurysm, microdialysis of glutamate was performed in order to monitor local metabolic changes in the medial temporal (all patients) and subfrontal cortex (four patients). The preliminary results indicate that: (i) extracellular glutamate concentrations may rise to very high levels after SAH and aneurysm surgery, (ii) the increased levels of excitatory amino acids correlate with the clinical course, and (iii) a rise in extracellular glutamate in one region is not necessarily paralleled with a rise in the other, as seen by the simultaneous sampling from two different vascular territories.

Keywords: Aneurysmal subarachnoid haemorrhage; glutamate; intracerebral microdialysis; ischemia.

Introduction

Aneurysmal subarachnoid haemorrhage (SAH) is a cerebrovascular event with high morbidity and mortality, where the major causes of poor outcome are the effects of the initial bleed, surgical complications, and delayed ischemic deterioration (DID) due to cerebral vasospasm [8]. A possibility of monitoring cerebral metabolic changes continuously over time might be of clinical value, particularly during the period with increased risk for DID. So far, transcranial Doppler velocities, measured from the basal large conducting arteries, have been used to predict and verify DID in SAH patients. However, since disturbances in the microcirculation may not always be reflected in velocity changes in the large arteries, more sophisticated measures would be desirable in order to monitor local metabolic changes in areas affected by ischemia.

Of particular importance for ischemia and ischemic neuronal damage are the excitatory amino acid neurotransmitters, such as glutamate and aspartate [2]. Elevations of the extracellular glutamate concentration during ischemia may induce overstimulation of glutamate receptors eventually leading to neuronal death. The intracerebral microdialysis technique [10] has been adopted to study neurotransmitter release, including glutamate, and animal experiments have shown that extracellular glutamate levels increase dramatically in the brain during ischemia [1,3].

We have used microdialysis of glutamate to study local ischemic events in seven patients with aneurysmal SAH [9]. Since vasospasm is rarely a global cerebral phenomenon but rather restricted to a single vascular territory, four of the patients had probes implanted both in the medial temporal and subfrontal cortex.

Materials and Methods

At the end of aneurysm surgery (1–2 days after the bleed), a sterilized microdialysis probe (obtained from the Department of Anatomy and Cell Biology, University of Gothenburg) with an outer diameter of 0.9 mm and 8 mm of dialysis membrane (Cuprophan B4AH) was inserted by free hand 1.5 cm into the tip of the gyrus temporalis superior (all patients) and into the gyrus subfrontalis (patients 4–7) ipsilateral to the aneurysm. Each probe was secured by suturing the tube to the dura and scalp. Sampling was started the following day by connecting the probe inlet to a microinfusion system (CMA Microdialysis, Stockholm). Sterile 0.9% saline was perfused at a rate of $2 \, \mu l/min$. In patients 4–7, dialysis was performed during day-time with the probe disconnected from the pump between sessions. The first 60 min perfusate was discarded at each sampling period. Dialysis was discontinued when the patient was fully mobilised, or for technical reasons. After removing the catheters from the patient, they were tested for in vitro recovery, which was $2.7 \pm 0.2\%$ for glutamate at room temperature.

The dialysates were analysed for glutamate using reversed-phase high-performance liquid chromatography with pre-column *o*-phthaldialdehyde derivatization [4]. The reported levels were not corrected for recovery.

Results

Patient 1. This 39 year-old man, who suffered from SAH-associated intracerebral hematoma caused by a ruptured middle cerebral artery (MCA) aneurysm, was comatose on admission and during the dialysis period (38–69 hours after ictus). Levels of glutamate from the medial temporal lobe were on average 12 μM without major variations. He ended up with a right-sided hemiparesis and dysphasia.

Patient 2. 64-year-old woman who had bled from an anterior communicating artery (ACoA) aneurysm. Medial temporal glutamate levels (63–93 hours after the bleed) averaged 0.6 μM. She was in good clinical condition throughout the treatment period and recovered without neurological sequelae.

Patient 3. Glutamate levels (61–94 hours after ictus) from the medial temporal lobe were low also in this patient (0.3 μM), who had an internal carotid artery (ICA) aneurysm. She had no symptoms of DID and made a good recovery.

Patient 4. This 38 year-old female, who had bled from a MCA aneurysm, was drowsy on admission. Glutamate levels were relatively low (<1 μM) during the first day of dialysis (71–84 hours post-ictus) both in samples from the temporal lobe and the subfrontal cortex. However, during the following days (100–175 hours after ictus) the levels increased, particularly in the temporal lobe where they reached on average 8.2 μM 125 hours after the bleed (corresponding levels in the subfrontal cortex were 1.3 μM). During the period of increased glutamate levels, the patient demonstrated signs of DID with dysphasia and increased transcranial Doppler velocities in the MCA.

Patient 5. This 50 year-old female who suffered from a ruptured ICA aneurysm, was in good clinical condition during the study period and made an uneventful recovery. She displayed higher glutamate levels in the subfrontal compared to the medial temporal cortex during the two dialysis sessions (approx. 72 and 97 hours after the bleed), with values of 5.4 and 8.9 μM subfrontally and 2.6 and 2.1 μM temporally, respectively.

Patient 6. This 49 year-old female was comatose on admission after a massive SAH from a ruptured ACoA aneurysm. Very high levels of glutamate (32.8 μM) were sampled from the subfrontal cortex 75 hours after the bleed, whereas temporal levels were only 2.8 μM. The next day, the glutamate levels were reduced markedly in both regions (2.3 μM subfrontally and 0.8 μM temporally). The patient finally ended up with severe cognitive sequelae.

Patient 7. This 40 year-old female suffered from a ruptured ACoA aneurysm and was in good clinical condition on admission and during the first two days of dialysis (up to 70 hours post-ictus). Glutamate levels were initially high in the subfrontal cortex (5.0 μM) but declined to below 1 μM the next day. However, at 94 and 117 hours after ictus subfrontal glutamate levels increased to 4.8 and 5.8 μM, respectively. These elevated levels coincided with confusion and later the patient developed a monoparesis. Temporal levels of glutamate were <1 μM throughout the study period.

Discussion

The present preliminary results show that extracellular glutamate concentrations in the subfrontal and medial temporal cortex can reach high levels in patients with SAH and also that the observed levels may correlate with the patient's clinical status. Firstly, patients 1 and 6 who initially were in a poor condition, demonstrated the highest glutamate levels (12 and 33 μM) and ended up with severe neurological sequelae. By contrast, glutamate levels in the medial temporal lobe were below 1.5 μM in patients 2 and 3 who were in good condition and had an uneventful clinical course. Secondly, the DID observed in patients 4 and 7 was paralleled with increased glutamate levels in the correlating vascular territory. Thus, increased levels of glutamate were recorded in the temporal lobe of patient 4 during the period of dysphasia, and in the subfrontal lobe of patient 7 who became confused. This also indicates that excessive glutamate release may be restricted to very localized vascular regions and that the position of the microdialysis probe is of critical importance for the interpretation of the results.

Brain ischemia is known to result in several physiological responses that depend on the severity of the ischemic insult [6]. Blood flow below 10–15% of control values has been shown to induce increased extracellular glutamate release [5] probably due to ischemia-induced shortage of ATP which stimulates glutamate release and inhibits glutamate reuptake [7]. The high levels of glutamate measured in some of the patients in the present study would, therefore, indicate severe ischemia and a risk for ischemic neuronal damage [2].

For the future, bedside analysis of excitatory amino acids with an on-line system may be of value for detecting ongoing ischemic events and may enable optimized treatment. The use of drugs that interfere with glutamatergic neurotransmission may be of particular interest in this respect.

References

1. Benveniste H, Drejer J, Schousboe A, Diemer NH (1984) Elevation of the extracellular concentrations of glutamate and aspartate in rat hippocampus during transient cerebral ischemia monitored by intracerebral microdialysis. J Neurochem 43: 1369–1374
2. Choi DW (1988) Glutamate neurotoxicity and disease of the nervous system. Neuron 1: 623–634
3. Hillered L, Hallström Å, Segersvärd S, Persson L, Ungerstedt U (1990) Dynamics of extracellular metabolites in the striatum after middle cerebral artery occlusion in the rat monitored by intracerebral microdialysis. J Cereb Blood Flow Metab 10: 149–151
4. Lindroth P, Mopper K (1979) High performance liquid chromatographic determination of subpicomole amounts of amino acids by precolumn fluorescence derivatization with o-phthaldialdehyde. Anal Chem 51: 127–132
5. Shimada N, Graf R, Rosner G, Wakayama A, George CP, Heiss W-D (1989) Ischemic flow thresholds for extracellular glutamate increase in cerebral cortex. J Cereb Blood Flow Metab 9: 603–606
6. Siesjö BK, Bengtsson F (1989) Calcium fluxes, calcium antagonists and calcium related pathology in brain ischemia, hypoglycemia and spreading depression; a unifying hypothesis. J Cereb Blood Flow Metab 9: 127–140
7. Szatkowski M, Attwell D (1994) Triggering and execution of neuronal death in brain ischemia: two phases of glutamate release by different mechanisms. Trends Neurosci 17: 359–365
8. Säveland H, Hillman J, Brandt L, Edner G, Jakobsson K-E, Algers G (1992) Overall outcome in aneurysmal subarachnoid hemorrhage. A prospective study from neurosurgical units in Sweden during a 1-year period. J Neurosurg 76: 729–734
9. Säveland H, Nilsson OG, Boris-Möller F, Wieloch T, Brandt L (1995) Intracerebral microdialysis of glutamate and aspartate in two vascular territories after aneurysmal subarachnoid hemorrhage. Neurosurgery 38: 12–20
10. Ungerstedt U (1984) Measurement of neurotransmitter release by intracranial dialysis. In: Marsden CA (ed) Measurements of neurotransmitter release in vivo. Wiley, New York, pp 81–105

Correspondence: O.G. Nilsson, M.D., Ph.D., Department of Neurosurgery, Lund University Hospital, S-221 85 Lund, Sweden.

Acta Neurochir (1996) [Suppl] 67: 48–52
© Springer-Verlag 1996

Microdialytic Monitoring of the Cortex During Neurovascular Surgery

A. Mendelowitsch[1], **H. Langemann**[2], **B. Alessandri**[2], **A. Kanner**[1], **H. Landolt**[3], and **O. Gratzl**[1]

[1]University Neurosurgical Clinic, [2]Section of Neurosurgery, Department of Research, Cantonal Hospital, Basel, Switzerland, and
[3]Neurosurgical Clinic, Cantonal Hospital, Aarau, Switzerland

Summary

Using microdialysis combined with suitable analytical methods, levels of metabolites in the extracellular fluid of the cerebral cortex were monitored during neurovascular surgery (9 aneurysm and 5 bypass operations). Our aim was to use microdialysis to detect any local ischaemia which could be caused by brain retraction, temporary clipping and dissecting manoevres. For this purpose, parameters were quantified whose levels in the dialysate are known to be influenced by ischaemia (on-line pH, ascorbic acid, uric acid, glutathione, cysteine, glucose, lactate). In the aneurysm series, the on-line pH fell after introduction of the retractor, and rose after removal; also, in many cases, levels of ascorbic acid, glutathione and lactate increased and glucose decreased. These changes are all in accordance with ischaemic conditions in the region of the probe; they disappeared at the end of retraction, or sometimes even before. During the bypass operations, there were no marked changes in on-line pH or in any of the measured parameters. However, in 2 of these patients ascorbic acid, uric acid and glucose levels were very high during the whole measurement, indicating possible changes in metabolism caused by inadequate perfusion (carotid artery stenosis). We conclude that microdialysis is a sensitive method of detecting intraoperative changes in cerebral metabolism.

Keywords: Microdialysis; cerebral ischaemia; retraction; EC-IC bypass.

Introduction

Neurovascular surgery e.g. for aneurysm or extracranial-intracranial (EC-IC) bypass, entails a number of procedures which might be associated with ischaemic conditions. For instance, it is known that self-retaining brain retractors, as required for adequate exposure during aneurysm operations, can cause local ischaemia [1]. Local ischaemic damage could be caused during temporary clipping of blood vessels for bypass procedures. Additionally, most EC-IC patients suffer from unilateral carotid occlusion, which is usually accompanied by reduced perfusion of the aff- ected hemisphere. This, depending on the collateral circulation, might lead to chronic ischaemic changes in the cortex. Monitoring of retractor blade pressure, brain electrical activity and cerebral blood flow can provide information about physiological parameters during retraction [1]. However, there is not yet any direct evidence of concomitant ischaemic changes in brain metabolism during a neurovascular operation.

Microdialysis is a method which has been widely used to demonstrate neurochemical changes in animal models of ischaemia, and which has been shown to be feasible intraoperatively [4, 9]. Changes of levels in the extracellular fluid (ECF) of various biochemical parameters can be continuously monitored. Parameters whose ECF levels have been shown to be influenced by ischaemic conditions include pH [6], glucose [8], lactate [3], glutamate [3], and the antioxidants ascorbic acid (Asc), glutathione (GSH), cysteine (Cys) and uric acid (UA) [2, 5].

In this study we have used microdialysis to monitor metabolism in the cerebral cortex during aneurysm and EC-IC bypass operations, using the above mentioned parameters. The aim was to see if any ischaemic changes could be detected and quantified during such operations.

Methods

Measurements were carried out during nine operations for aneurysm of the carotid circulation, all needing frontal retraction. One patient (D.Sch.) had 2 aneurysms, only one of which required use of a retractor. Patient H.L. underwent a tumour operation without retraction before clipping of the aneurysm. Five extra-intracranial (EC-IC) bypass operations (2 in the same patient with an interval of 4 months) were also monitored.

Immediately after the craniotomy, before opening the dura, a 1 cm cut was made in the dura and the probe (4 mm membrane, 0.5 mm diameter), which had been previously sterilised at 60°C with ethylene dioxide, was inserted into the cortex (for the aneurysm operation, frontally; for the bypass, temporally 1–1.5 cm from the bypass site). In patient K.K., in whom a temporal retractor was also needed, a second probe was placed in the temporal lobe. The probes were perfused with sterile 0.9% saline at 2 µl/min (in one bypass operation, 4 µl/min) until the dura was closed. Fractions of 40 or 50 µl were collected. During most operations the on-line pH of the dialysate was recorded [6]. After the end of the operation, the in vitro relative recoveries for all parameters were measured at room temperature using the same probe, flow rate and perfusion medium as in the operation. Relative recovery is defined as the ratio (%) between the concentration of a substance in the perfusion outflow to that of the same substance in the solution surrounding the probe. Asc, UA, GSH, and Cys were determined in the dialysate (5 µl) by reverse phase HPLC and electrochemical detection with a gold electrode (0.65 V). Glucose was determined colorimetrically in 15 µl or 20 µl using a kit (Trinder from Sigma). Lactate was determined by an enzymatic fluorimetric method, also in 15 µl or 20 µl. In one case glutamate was also measured by HPLC, after derivatisation with phenyl isothiocyanate.

Results

Aneurysm Operations

Asc was increased in 6 patients during retraction, as was GSH in 7 patients. In two cases both parameters showed considerable increases, of up to 7-fold for Asc and 15-fold for GSH, whereas in the others increases were smaller. Basal levels of Cys were not generally measurable; however this parameter could be detected in 2 patients during retraction. Lactate was increased in 5 patients, with a concomitant fall in glucose. In all patients, values of parameters returned almost to the original levels, often before the end of retraction. Figure 1 shows the time course of microdialysis in patient H.L. During tumour removal, baseline conditions were observed. Subsequently the retractor was placed to enable aneurysm clipping, and immediate changes in all the detectable parameters (except glucose) could be noted.

In the patient with two probes (K.K.), frontal effects were much greater than temporal ones for all measured parameters (see Fig. 2). The two probes used had similar recovery characteristics (Asc, 11% and 10%; UA, 21% and 19%; glucose, 29% and 30%; lactate, 18% and 17%, for frontal and temporal probes respectively).

In one patient, D. Sch., glutamate values were measured. As can be seen in Fig. 3, there was a marked rise in glutamate during and after retraction, with a subsequent slow return to a basal level of about 7.6 µM during the latter part of the operation, when no retrac-

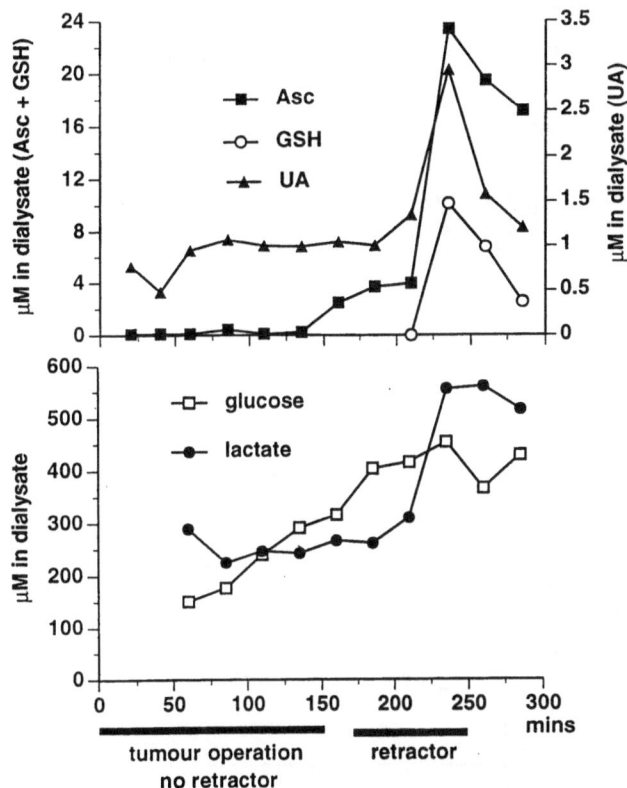

Fig. 1. Cortical microdialysis during a tumour operation and aneurysm surgery in patient H.L. Ascorbic acid (*Asc*), uric acid (*UA*), glutathione (*GSH*), glucose and lactate were detected in the dialysate

tor was needed. Figure 4 shows changes in on-line pH for this patient. Values fell nearly 0.3 units during retraction, with a return to a steady basal level of about 6.93 afterwards. Similar reductions in on-line pH were observed in the other patients during retraction.

Average values (mean ± s.e.m, n = 9) for the last sample collected before closure of the dura (for patient H.L., last sample before use of the retractor) were as follows: Asc, 5.8 ± 1.1 µM; UA, 5.0 ± 1.6 µM; glucose, 266 ± 35 µM; lactate, 239 ± 22 µM; pH 7.1 ± 0.1. Recoveries (n = 8) were: Asc, 12.1 ± 3.8%; UA, 21.1 ± 3.2%; glucose, 26.6 ± 4.8%; lacate, 20.9 ± 4.2%.

EC-IC Bypass

In the first 4 operations, there were no marked changes in values of the measured parameters, and on-line pH was not affected. As this bypass operation is rather short, the flow rate was increased from 2 µl to 4 µl in the last patient (W.S.), to enable the time interval between samples to be reduced to 10 min. During this operation, after the clipping, there was a temporary reduction of glucose down to unmeasurable values

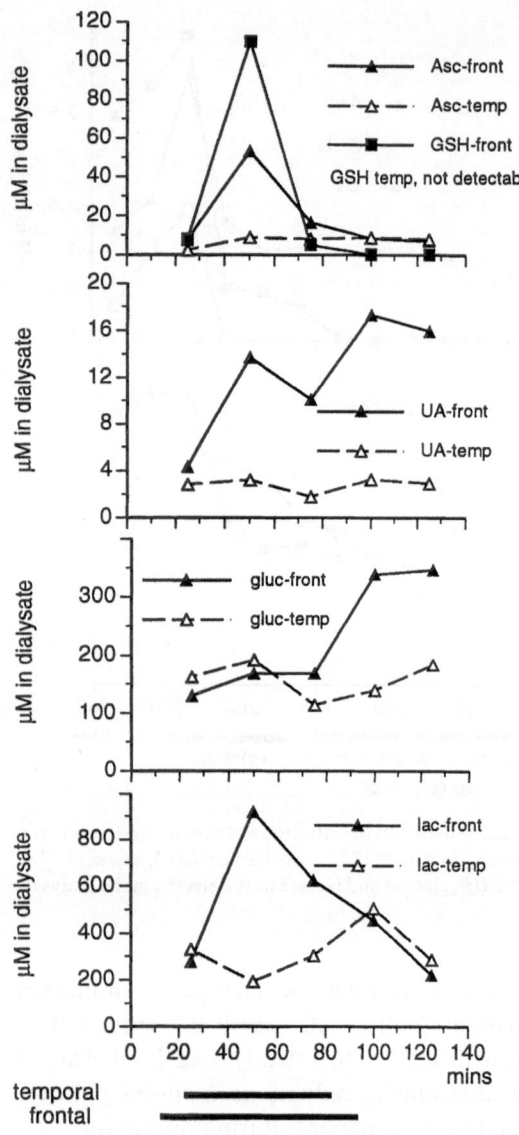

Fig. 2. Cortical microdialysis during aneurysm surgery in patient
K.K. One probe was inserted frontally (*front*) and another temporally (*temp*). Ascorbic acid (*Asc*), uric acid (*UA*), glutathione (*GSH*),
glucose (*gluc*) and lactate (*lac*) were detected in the dialysates

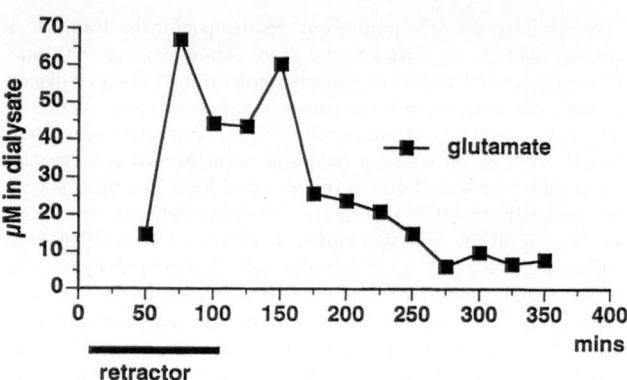

Fig. 3. Cortical microdialysis during aneurysm surgery in patient
D.Sch., showing changes in glutamate levels

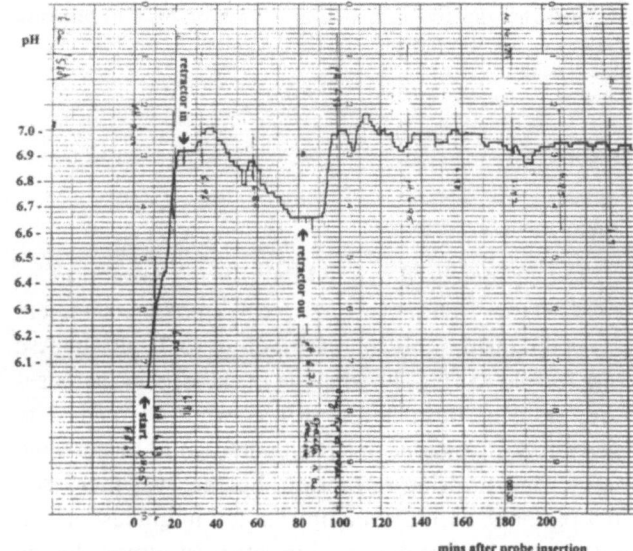

Fig. 4. Original trace showing changes in on-line pH of the cortical
dialysate during aneurysm surgery

during 20 minutes; this was not accompanied by any
increase in lactate. There was also a slight reduction in
pH. Average values found during these operations are
given in Table 1. In calculating the averages the first

Table 1. *Values of Parameters Obtained During EC-IC Bypass Operations*

Patient	n	Ascorbic acid	Uric acid	Glucose	Lactate	pH
		Mean (µM in dialysate) $\pm$ s.e.m.				
F.L. (r. side)	7	12.2 $\pm$ 0.7	19.3 $\pm$ 1.4	563 $\pm$ 59	166 $\pm$ 11	7.2–7.3
F.L. (l. side)	5	5.9 $\pm$ 0.7	2.3 $\pm$ 0.2	37 $\pm$ 5	102 $\pm$ 15	6.94–7.0
O.M.	5	15.4 $\pm$ 0.6	3.3 $\pm$ 0.2	267 $\pm$ 37	271 $\pm$ 26	6.9–7.18
L.E.	5	7.6 $\pm$ 1.1	13.9 $\pm$ 1.4	581 $\pm$ 59	206 $\pm$ 26	7.0–7.1
W.S.	5	7.6 $\pm$ 1.1	7.7 $\pm$ 0.9	159 $\pm$ 22	386 $\pm$ 52	6.76–7.03

n number of samples included in the evaluation; pH was measured on-line. For patient W.S., flow rate was 4 µl/min.

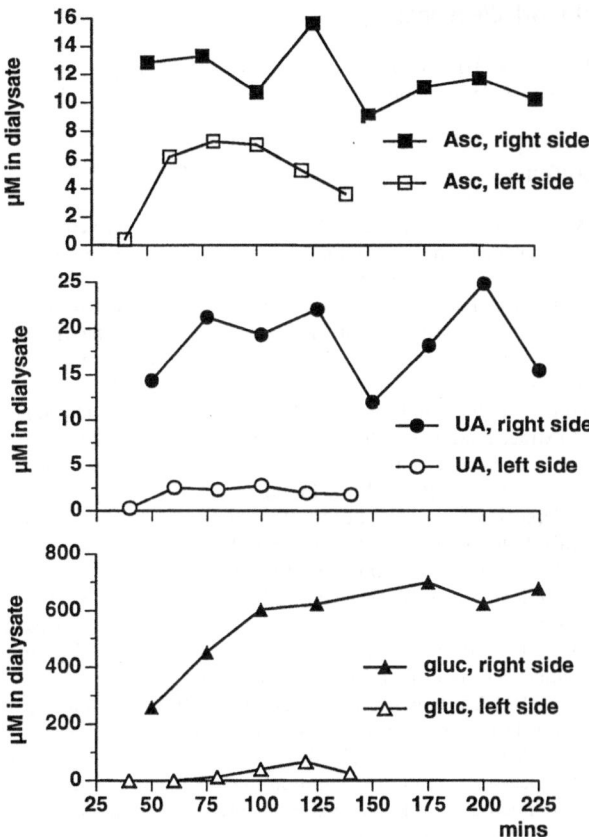

Fig. 5. Cortical microdialysis during 2 EC-IC bypass operations (left side 4 months after right side). Note that levels of ascorbic acid (*Asc*), uric acid (*UA*) and glucose (*gluc*) are higher on the right side, although relative recoveries were similar in the 2 probes

samples were omitted, as stable conditions had not been reached.

Patient F.L. was operated on the right side for complete carotid stenosis, and 4 months later on the left side for partial carotid stenosis. We were able to monitor both operations. The results are shown in Fig. 5. It can be seen that values of Asc, UA and glucose are very much higher during the first operation (right side) than during the second, although recoveries of the two probes used were in the same range (Asc, 9.9% and 13.3%; UA, 23% and 32%; lactate, 10% and 16%; glucose 15% and 10%, for right side and left side respectively). These values of Asc, UA and glucose are also higher than those in aneurysm patients (see above). Similar elevated values were found in another bypass patient.

Discussion

In this study we have confirmed that microdialysis is a sensitive tool for detecting metabolic changes in-

traoperatively. In most of our patients retraction was followed by neurochemical changes similar to those obtained during ischaemic events, i.e. increases in dialysate levels of Asc, lactate, GSH and cysteine, reduction in on-line pH, and reduction in dialysate glucose (Figs. 1 and 2). Glutamate, which was only measured in one patient, also increased during retraction (Fig. 3). Corresponding changes in all these parameters have been found in microdialysates from the ischaemic zone of rats subjected to middle cerebral artery occlusion [2, 3, 5, 6]. In addition, similar results were found in microdialysates from a patient with severe head injury, where there was practically no cerebral perfusion [7]. However, changes during retraction were temporary, and were not found in all patients. In every case they returned more or less rapidly to the initial values, sometimes even before the end of retraction. This may be because retraction was routinely intermittent with frequent changes of position. Moreover, animal experiments have shown that the brain accomodates itself rapidly to retraction pressure (monitored retraction pressure dropped to 50% of its original value after 6–12 mins) [1]. Neurological and postoperative CT findings did not indicate ischaemic changes frontally in any of the patients.

The results from patient K.K. (Fig. 2) where two probes were implanted, one frontally and one temporally, showed that the changes of levels in the dialysates were not artefacts, but were related to the duration and pressure of retraction, factors which were both less temporally than frontally.

On-line pH measurement is of special interest as it provides information from the cortex of the patient with a time-lag of only 12–18 min (variable, depending on the length of the tubing from the probe to the pH meter). However, in one patient, there was a decrease in pH (to 6.78) during 90 mins of retraction, followed by a rapid unexpected increase of pH to 7.31. Later we found greatly increased UA and glucose in the fractions collected during and after the pH rise. The patient recovered normally, but a routine postoperative CT showed a tiny haemorrhage near to the probe insertion point. Thus, the increase in pH and other changes can probably be explained by the presence of blood in the ECF. This finding indicates that care must be taken in the interpretation of data from cerebral microdialysis.

Because of our interest in cerebral monitoring in trauma patients, we wanted to get an idea of basal levels of our parameters in dialysates from minimally disturbed brain. Values before operation were not available, as the interval between probe insertion and application of the retractor was usually too short for equilibrium to be reached. However, in the patient with two probes, levels in the last fraction before probe removal were similar frontally and temporally although the severity of the retractor insult had differed greatly (Fig. 2). We can therefore assume that levels in these fractions approximate to the above-mentioned basal levels. The values for Asc, GSH and lactate are similar to those found by us [7] and other authors [4].

Our aims in monitoring the EC-IC bypass operations were twofold. Besides looking for ischaemic changes during clipping procedures, we wanted to find out if the chronically reduced blood supply to the hemisphere affected by carotid occlusion had had any detectable effect on the cerebral metabolism. As CBF and SPECT measurements after bypass operations show an improvement in many patients, there might also be changes after performing the operation.

Results showed that there were generally no acute ischaemic changes similar to those occurring during retraction, in an EC-IC bypass operation. It could be that the microdialysis probe was situated outside the territory of the small branch of the medial cerebral artery which was clipped.

On the other hand, in two of the patients levels of glucose, ascorbic acid and uric acid were much higher than in the aneurysm patients at the end of the operation. One example of this can be seen in Fig. 5, right side, whereas levels on the left side were in the range of those found in the aneurysm patients. The significance of these increased values remains to be investigated.

Acknowledgements

We thank Mrs. V. Jäggin Verin, Basel, for carrying out the glutamate determination.

References

1. Andrews RJ, Bringas JR (1993) A review of brain retraction and recommendation for minimizing intraoperative brain injury. Neurosurgery 33: 1052–1064
2. Hillered L, Persson L, Bolander HG, Hallström A, Ungerstedt U (1988) Increased extracellular levels of ascorbate in the striatum after middle cerebral artery occlusion in the rat monitored by intracerebral microdialysis. Neurosci Lett 95: 286–290
3. Hillered L, Persson L, Ponten U, Ungerstedt U (1989) Dynamics of extracellular metabolites in the striatum after middle cerebral artery occlusion in the rat monitored by intracerebral microdialysis. J Cereb Blood Flow Metab 9: 607–616
4. Hillered L, Persson L, Pontén U, Ungerstedt U (1990) Neurometabolic monitoring of the ischemic human brain using microdialysis. Acta Neurochir (Wien) 102: 91–97
5. Landolt H, Lutz TW, Langemann H, Stäuble D, Mendelowitsch A, Gratzl O (1992) Extracellular antioxidants and amino acids in the cortex of the rat: monitoring by microdialysis of early ischemic changes. J Cereb Blood Flow Metab 12: 96–102
6. Landolt H, Langemann H, Gratzl O (1993) On-line monitoring of cerebral pH using microdialysis. Neurosurgery 32: 1000–1004
7. Landolt H, Langemann H, Mendelowitsch A, Gratzl O (1994) Neurochemical monitoring and on-line pH measurements using brain microdialysis in patients in intensive care. Acta Neurochir (Wien) [Suppl] 60: 475–478
8. Langemann H, Mendelowitsch A, Landolt H, Alessandri B, Gratzl O (1995) Experimental and clinical monitoring of glucose by microdialysis. Clin Neurol Neurosurg 97: 149–155
9. Mendelowitsch A, Langemann H, Landolt H, Gratzl O (1994) Microdialytic monitoring of ischemic changes during brain retraction for aneurysm surgery. In: Nagai H *et al* (eds) Intracranial pressure IX. Springer, Berlin Heidelberg New York Tokyo, pp 260–263

Correspondence: A Mendelowitsch, M.D., Neurosurgical Clinic, Kantonsspital, CH-4031 Basel, Switzerland.

Acta Neurochir (1996) [Suppl] 67: 53–58
© Springer-Verlag 1996

In-vivo Microdialysis Study of Extracellular Glutamate Response to Temperature Variance in Subarachnoid Hemorrhage

A. Shuaib, R. Kanthan, G. Goplen, R. Griebel, H. El-Azzouni, H. Miyashita, L. Liu, and **T. Hogan**

Department of Medicine (Neurology), Surgery (Neurosurgery), Community Health and Epidemiology and the Saskatchewan Stroke Research Centre, Royal University Hospital, Saskatoon, SK, Canada

Summary

Neurochemical changes may precede the development of clinical signs in neurological disease. Early identification of such changes may offer an opportunity to avoid or treat complications. Under experimental conditions, extracellular levels of glutamate and other amino acids can be monitored by in-vivo microdialysis in cerebral ischemia, head trauma and epilepsy. Data on the release of glutamate under ischemic conditions in humans are limited. There is no published data on the effects of temperature variation or other manipulations on the extracellular glutamate levels in humans. We report for the first time, the effects of changes in temperature on the extracellular cerebral glutamate levels as measured by in-vivo microdialysis, the dialysate being collected before, during and after cooling in four patients with subarachnoid hemorrhage. Three of the patients had in-vivo microdialysis carried out postoperatively. One patient underwent microdialysis three days prior to the surgical clipping of the aneurysm. In all patients, mild head cooling resulted in a significant decrease in extracellular glutamate levels. The effect of cooling was most apparent when the extracellular glutamate concentrations were high. In two patients, the extracellular glutamate levels increased sharply with fever but returned to normal once the temperature normalized. In vivo microdialysis can be used to measure extracellular glutamate and other neurotransmitters with minimal discomfort in awake humans. This technique offers a unique opportunity to monitor the neurochemistry in critically ill patients and it may aid in developing therapeutic intervention strategies to minimize undesired chemical responses.

Keywords: In-vivo microdialysis; glutamate; SAH; cooling; fever.

Introduction

Accurate information on the status of cerebral metabolism may be useful in the development of strategies to prevent brain damage during ischemia and other cerebral insults. Accessing the brain directly has proven difficult because of the thick skull bone. Monitoring with electroencephalography, computed tomography and magnetic resonance tomography offers little information on the biochemical derangements that may develop during disease. Positron emission tomography (PET) and MR spectroscopy though useful, have their limitations. An early identification of biochemical derangements may aid in the identification of subtle cerebral dysfunctions, which in turn would alert the physician to develop therapeutic interventions to abort such responses.

In-vivo microdialysis is a new technique that can directly study the extracellular neurochemistry in living subjects. It is in use in awake and anesthetized animals to study the effects of ischemia on the cerebral neurochemistry [1, 4, 6, 20, 28]. The technique has recently been used in patients with epilepsy [8, 22], in one patient with grade V subarachnoid hemorrhage and in patients with severe head trauma [20].

Vasospasm and rebleeding are the most serious complications of subarachnoid hemorrhage (SAH) [19]. Severe vasospasm can result in tissue hypoxia and cerebral infarction [19]. Cerebral angiography and transcranial Doppler (TCD) are the standard tests in use to detect vasospasm [19]. These techniques do not provide any information on tissue ischemia. In-vivo microdialysis and on-line neurochemical analysis may be a key tool to monitor chemical responses to acute ischemia. Such techniques may also be useful to monitor the response to therapeutic interventions.

We present our observations in four patients with SAH who underwent four hours of continuous in-vivo microdialysis on four consecutive days. These patients had changes in extracellular glutamate levels associated with mild head cooling recorded over these four days.

Patients and Methods

This study was approved by the University Advisory Committee on Ethics in Human Experimentation. Informed consent was obtained prior to the commencement of the study from the patients or their next of kin.

Case Reports

Patient no. 1: This patient complained of a sudden onset of headache and stiffness of the neck. A cranial CT scan showed SAH and a cerebral angiography confirmed an anterior communicating artery aneurysm. The aneurysm was clipped within 24 hours. At the same time a Codman bolt was inserted over the left frontal cortex for microdialysis monitoring. Microdialysis was commenced two hours after completion of surgery. The microdialysis probe was removed after 4 hours of collection. Daily microdialysis was carried out over the next four consecutive days. The patient was awake during the procedure. An angiogram performed four days after the surgery showed no evidence of vasospasm. The dialysate glutamate levels and the associated response to cooling are shown in Fig. 1.

Patient no. 2: This patient presented with a severe headache of sudden onset. Neurological examination was normal except for a mild neck stiffness. SAH was suspected and a lumbar puncture showed a bloody C.S.F. The patient was transferred to the Royal University Hospital and a CT scan confirmed SAH. Cerebral angiography on the same day showed a posterior communicating

artery aneurysm. This was surgically clipped within twenty-four hours of the ictal event and a Codman bolt inserted over the right frontal cortex for intracerebral microdialysis as in Patient 1. The dialysate glutamate levels and the associated response to cooling are shown in Fig. 2.

Patient no. 3: This patient developed a sudden onset of headache with a stiff neck. A cranial CT scan revealed a massive SAH. The source of the hemorrhage was not traceable on the first two cerebral angiograms performed two weeks apart. A third angiogram done four weeks later showed a saccular aneurysm of the internal carotid artery. The aneurysm was clipped and a Codman bolt inserted over the right frontal lobe after completion of surgery. In-vivo microdialysis was begun three days after the ictal event and continued for three days. The dialysate glutamate levels and the associated response to cooling are shown in Fig. 3.

Patient no. 4: This patient developed a sudden headache and rapidly lost consciousness. Examination showed the patient to be deeply comatose with marked neck stiffness. A cranial CT scan showed a large SAH with ventricular hemorrhage. Over the next five days he remained deeply comatose with a gradual improvement in clinical status. Microdialysis was done for three days beginning three days after the ictal event through a Codman bolt inserted over the right frontal cortex. The dialysate glutamate levels and the associated response to cooling are shown in Fig. 4.

The postoperative course in Patients 1, 2 and 3 was smooth and uneventful except for the onset of fever in Patients 2 and 3. They were all alert and awake during the recordings. The post operative CAT scans done on days 1 and 7 showed no unexpected findings. The post operative angiograms were satisfactory. The clinical outcome was good in Patient 1 and 2 with no residual deficits. Patient 3 suffered a clinical setback with the onset of pulmonary embolism. Neurologically, she had a mild residual paresis that gradually improved. Patient 4 improved from a Glasgow Coma scale of 4 to 8 during the 3 days of recording.

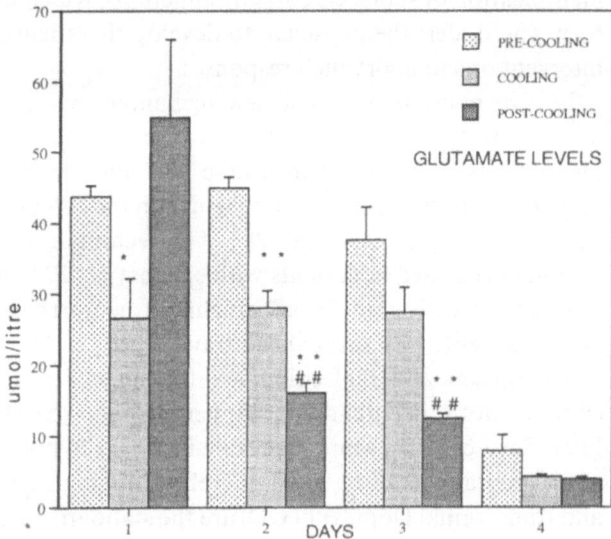

Fig. 1. Extracellular glutamate levels over four days in patient 1. The data represent a mean of six 10 minute collections and the bars are ±S.E.M. There are three sets of data per day. The data represent dialysate levels before (PRE-COOLING), during (COOLING) and after (POST-COOLING) cooling. There was a significant fall in the glutamate levels with head cooling in collections obtained on day 1, 2 and 3. On day 1 the glutamate levels increased upon removal of the stimulus. On days 2 and 3, the glutamate levels continued to fall after removal of cooling. On the final day of monitoring, the glutamate levels had fallen below 10 μmols/L and there was no significant decrease in glutamate levels with cooling. * p < 0.05, ** p < 0.01 (pre-cooling vs cooling and post cooling). # p < 0.05, ## p < 0.01 (pre-cooling vs post cooling), MANOVA (repeated measures) was used. Similar statistical analyses apply for all the figures

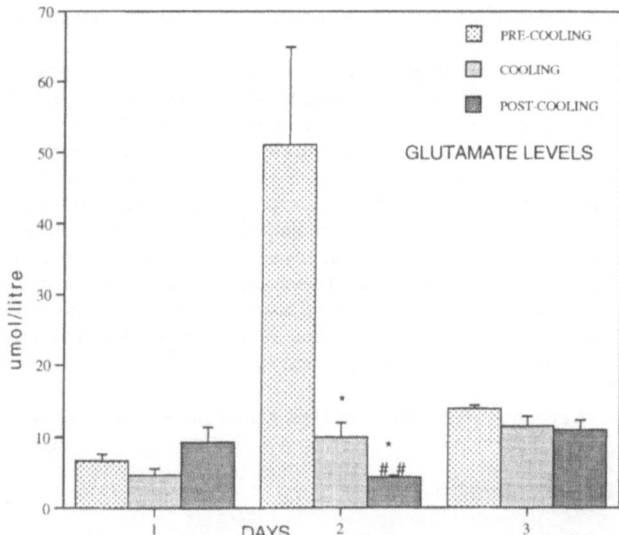

Fig. 2. The glutamate levels were very low on day 1 in the second patient. On the second day the patient was febrile. The initial collections prior to cooling reflect an increase in the extracellular glutamate that decreased significantly with head cooling. The decrease in glutamate levels continued even after the removal of the cooling hat. On the third day the glutamate levels were low and did not fall with head cooling

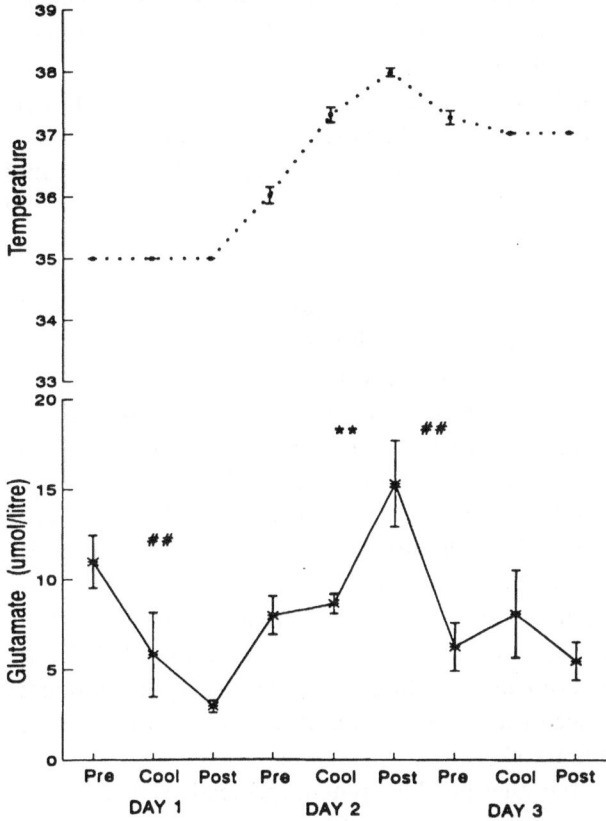

Fig. 3. The third patient was hypothermic on day 1. The patient developed a pulmonary embolus on the second day resulting in an increase in systemic temperature. Microdialysis collections of the second day show a significant increase in dialysate glutamate levels with a significant response to mild head cooling. On the third day, the temperature had returned to normal. Extracellular glutamate levels were low with no associated response to cooling

Methods

Microdialysis: We used custom-designed CMA/10 (Stockholm, Sweden) probes for all the analyses. Microdialysis was carried out by the "closed method" as described in our previous work [13]. Briefly, sterile Ringer's solution is used as in other in-vivo studies of the human brain [12, 17, 20] at an infusion rate of 2 microlitres per minute through a CMA-100 (Stockholm Sweden) pump. The fluid was collected on ice and immediately transferred for HPLC analysis. Collections over the initial one hour after probe insertion were discarded as implantation trauma may result in elevated levels of neurotransmitters. The fluid was collected in 10 minute segments. After 60 minutes (6 samples) of collection which served as the "baseline" a cooling hat (Manson and Manson Engineering, Longview WA) was placed on the head. The hats remained in place for approximately one hour. Six dialysate specimens were collected in these "cooled" conditions. The hats were subsequently removed and microdialysis was continued for a further 60 minutes before removal of the probes. This procedure was repeated for four consecutive days with new sterile probes every day. In between the analyses, the Codman bolt was kept locked. The patients were awake during most of the collections and tolerated the procedure without any complications.

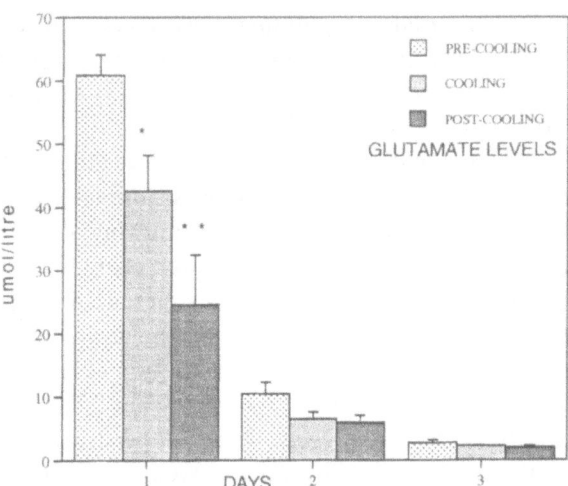

Fig. 4. This figure shows data from the fourth patient. This patient was comatose at the time of analyses. On day 1, the glutamate levels were high and responded well to cooling. On subsequent days, the glutamate levels had fallen below 10 μmols/L and did not respond to head cooling

HPLC analysis: The microdialysis fluid was analyzed for amino acids using HPLC and electrochemical detection. Measurements were done according to the methods of Donzani and Yamamoto [7] as previously described in detail with O-pthalaldehyde (OPA)/2-mercaptoethanol (BME) prior to detection with a 715 Ultra Wisp Sample Processor (Waters, Toronto, Canada). A Baseline Workstation Data Processing System (Waters, Toronto Canada) was used for data storage and analyses. The mobile phase consisted of di-sodium hydrogen orthophosphate 0.10 M, ethylenediaminetetraacetic acid di sodium salt 0.13 mM and methanol 28%. Standards of 0.625, 1.25, 2.5, 25, 100, 300 and 600 picomoles were used in all analyses. Each probe was checked for recovery at the end of the collection of samples. Temperature was recorded by the conventional oral route using a standard digital thermometer and hourly recordings were maintained during the microdialysis on all days.

Statistical analyses: Repeated measures MANOVA was used for the entire dataset for each patient and for individual day analysis between the pre-cooling (normothermic), cooling and post-cooling (hypothermic) collections. T-Test was used as a post-hoc test for within day comparisons. Bonfferoni correction technique was applied to the post-hoc test and thus a P value of 0.017 was used as the level of significance. Pearson's correlation analysis was carried out on Patient 2 and 3 on day 2 between the temperature recordings and the measured glutamate levels.

Results

The extracellular glutamate levels in the first patient are shown in Fig. 1. As can be seen from Fig. 1, there was a drop in the dialysate glutamate levels with the mild cooling on all four days. On day 1, dialysate glutamate levels reverted to higher levels when the hat was removed. On subsequent days, there was a further decline in extracellular glutamate concentrations once the hat was removed. The lower levels persisted until the end of the daily measurements. The reason for this decrease in the dialysate glutamate levels is not entirely clear. The dialysate glutamate levels however reverted to "baseline" levels at the start of the next day's collection on days 1, 2, and 3.

The second patient had low dialysate glutamate levels after surgery. These did not significantly decrease with cooling on the initial day of monitoring. On the second day the patient developed a fever, probably due to a systemic infection. The dialysate glutamate levels were high with this febrile episode (correlation coefficient r = 0.7682 (P = 0.0013). The initiation of cooling was associated with a rapid and significant fall in the extracellular glutamate levels. This effect persisted even when the cooling stimulus was removed. On the third day of collection, the patient's temperature had returned to normal. The dialysate glutamate concentrations were also low and failed to respond to cooling. The details of the associated extracellular glutamate response to cooling are shown in Fig. 2.

The third patient developed a fever on the second day of microdialysis. This was attributed to deep venous thrombosis complicated by a pulmonary embolism. The associated response to cooling was apparent on day 1. On day 2 the increase in body temperature was associated with an increase in the extracellular glutamate levels (r = 0.71452; p = 0.0019) despite the head cooling stimulus. Normal temperatures on day 3 were associated with low dialysate glutamate concentrations and little observed response to head cooling. The details of the rise in temperature and the corresponding changes in dialysate glutamate concentrations are depicted in Fig. 3.

The fourth patient was critically ill. Microdialysis was begun three days after the ictal event at a time when the aneurysm had not been clipped. The details of the dialysate glutamate levels and the response to cooling is shown in Fig. 4.

Discussion

We were able to detect extracellular glutamate levels by in-vivo microdialysis in all our patients. It was possible to monitor the associated response of these levels to changes in temperature with no added discomfort to the patients. Mild head cooling with a cooling hat was associated with a decrease in extracellular glutamate levels. A rise in temperature was associated with elevated extracellular glutamate levels. In-vivo microdialysis may be a useful tool to study the ongoing biochemical changes in the chemically "unstable" brain.

Cerebral ischemia results in a sudden severe increase in extracellular glutamate levels [1, 18]. These rapidly fall with reperfusion [1].

Brief insults result in a sudden increase in glutamate in contrast to a mild elevation with a more prolonged insult. The interruption of blood flow leads to a rapid loss of energy sources (ATP, etc.) and derangement of ion homeostasis [21, 26, 29]. This produces membrane depolarization and an increase in the extracellular glutamate [1, 9, 11]. The associated ion fluxes result in the intracellular accumulation of calcium [5]. This activates various intracellular lipolytic, proteolytic and nucleolytic enzyme systems which, if severe and prolonged, lead to irreversible cell injury [24, 25, 29]. The glutamate concentration inside the cells is approximately 10 µmol/L [15]. The normal extracellular mammalian glutamate concentration is 0.6 µmol/L. The baseline values in the temporal lobe of the human brain are 20.22 ± 3.39 µM as reported in our work on the ischemic model of the human brain [14]. Under experimental conditions, an increase in the glutamate concentrations by 2–5 µmol/L may result in neuronal damage [15].

Hypothermia has potent protective effects when used during ischemia [10, 16]. There is experimental evidence that mild hypothermia (1–3 degrees Celsius) may be neuroprotective when used during or immediately following an ischemic insult [2, 3, 23]. The mechanism for this protection is likely to be multifactorial and may include a decrease in extracellular glutamate (decreased release and/or increased re-uptake), diminished energy-metabolism and a slower intracellular build-up of calcium [10]. One of the mechanisms by which small variations in brain temperature exert their protective effect involves the reduction of ischemia-induced glutamate release [3]. In our patients, the extracellular glutamate concentrations were usually elevated in the post-surgical interval and with raised temperatures. The decrease in extracellular glutamate concentrations with the very mild hypothermia stimulus suggests that such an intervention may have a therapeutic potential. The efficacy of hypothermia in SAH is not evaluated in our study.

Direct measurement of brain temperature in humans is difficult and requires invasive techniques [10]. The core body temperature has a close relationship to brain temperature in awake individuals [10]. In patients with severe head-injury the brain temperature may be higher than the core temperature [10]. We were unable to monitor the brain temperature of our patients as they were awake and had no evidence of head injury. The core temperature should, therefore, reflect the brain temperature. We are also uncertain about the exact degree of hypothermia produced by the cooling hats. The changes were, in all likelihood, mild. However, even with this mild hypothermic stimulus, the decrease in extracellular glutamate concentrations was significant and persistent. Similarly, the associated increase in extracellular glutamate was very dramatic with a rise in temperature. These observations have important clinical implications. For potential clinical trials in stroke, head injury and post-cardiac arrest patients, we may not need a major drop in temperature to cause a lasting decrease in extracellular glutamate. The associated increase in extracellular glutamate with mild fever confirms our belief that change in temperature is an important variable and warrants close monitoring in an acute neurological setting. This is in keeping with MR studies in rats that have shown a marked increase in neuronal damage in hyperthermic animals in comparison to either the normothermic or the hypothermic group [27]. The possibility that mild hyperthermia can aggravate ischemic tissue injury necessitates prompt treatment of any rise in temperature in patients with subarachnoid hemorrhage who are at risk for ischemia [27]. Absence of direct brain temperature measurements is perhaps a major weakness of our study.

Based on our study of four patients with SAH we conclude that cooling of the head is associated with a decrease in dialysate glutamate levels. This response is marked when the extracellular glutamate levels are $> 40\,\mu M$. When the extracellular glutamate levels are $< 10\,\mu M$ this response is not observed. There is also a trend for the extracellular glutamate levels to increase with a rise in systemic temperature. The exact source of this extracellular glutamate is unknown. Whether it represents the general metabolic pool is speculative and thereby raises the question as to whether this is a true cellular increase or a reaccumulation phenomenon. These concepts, we feel, need further study.

References

1. Benveniste H, Dreger J, Schousboe A, Diemer NH (1984) Elevation of extracellular concentration of glutamate and asparate in rat hippocampus during transient cerebral ischemia monitored by intracerebral microdialysis. J Neurochem 43: 1369–1374
2. Busto RB, Dietrich D, Globus MY-T, Valdes I, Scheinberg P, Ginsberg MD (1987) Small differences in intraischemic temperatures critically determine the extent of ischemic neuronal injury. J Cereb Blood Flow Metab 7: 729–738
3. Busto R, Globus MYT, Dietrich WD, Martinez E, Valdes I, Ginsberg M (1989) Effects of mild hypothermia on ischemia-induced release of neurotransmitters and free fatty acids in rat brain. Stroke 20: 904–910
4. Carlson H, Ronne-Engström E, Ungerstedt U, Hillered (1992) Seizure related elevations of extracellular amino acids in human focal epilepsy. Neurosci Lett 140: 30–32
5. Choi DW (1988) Calcium-mediated neurotoxicity: relationship to specific channel types and role in ischemic damage. Trends Neurosci 11: 465–469
6. Di Chiara G (1990) In-vivo brain dialysis of neurotransmitters. Trends Phormacol Sci 11: 116–121
7. Donzanti BA, Yamamoto BK (1988) An improved and rapid HPLC-EC method for the isocratic separation of amino acid neurotransmitters from brain tissue and microdialysis perfusates. Life Sci 43: 913–922
8. During MJ, Spencer DD (1993) Extracellular hippocampal glutamate and spontaneous seizure in the conscious human brain. Lancet 341: 1607–1610
9. Garcia JH, Anderson ML (1989) Pathophysiology of cerebral ischemia. Crit Rev Neurobiol 4: 303–324
10. Ginsberg MD, Sternau LL, Globus MY-T, Dietrich WD, Busto R (1992) Therapeutic modulation of brain temperature: relevance to ischemic brain injury. Cerebrovasc Brain Metab Rev 4: 189–225
11. Globus MYT, Busto R, Dietrich WD, Martinez E, Valdes I, Ginsberg MD (1988) Effect of ischemia on the in-vivo release of striatal dopamine, glutamate, and y-aminobutyric acid studied by intracerebral microdialysis. J Neurochem 51: 1455–1464
12. Hillered L, Persson L, Ponten U, Ungerstedt U (1990) Neurometabolic monitoring of the ischemic human brain using microdialysis. Acta Neurochir (Wien) 102: 91–97
13. Kanthan R, Shuaib A, Goplen G, Miyashita H (1995) A new method of in-vivo microdialysis of the human brain. J Neursci Methods 60: 151–155
14. Kanthan R, Shuaib A, Griebel A, Miyashita H (1995) Intracerebral human microdialysis in vivo study of an acute focal ischemic model of the human brain. Stroke 26: 5
15. Lipton SA, Rosenberg PA (1994) Excitatory aminoacids as a final common pathway for neurologic disorders. N Engl J Med 330: 613–622
16. Maher J, Hachinski V (1993) Hypothermia as a potential treatment for cerebral ischemia. Cerebrovasc Brain Metab Rev 5: 277–300
17. Meyerson BA, Linderoth B, Karlsson H, Ungerstedt U (1990) Microdialysis in the human brain: extracellular measurements in the thalamus of Parkinsonian patients. Life Sci 46: 301–308
18. Mitani A, Andou Y, Kataoka K (1992) Selective vulnerability of hippocampal CA1 neurons cannot be explained in terms of an increase in glutamate concentration during ischemia in the gerbil: brain microdialysis study. Neuroscience 48: 307–313
19. Mohr JP, Kistler JP, Fink ME (1992) Intracranial aneurysms. In: Barnett HJ, Mohr JP, Stein BM, Yatsu FM (eds) Stroke: pathophysiology, diagnosis and management, 2nd Ed. Churchill Livingstone, New York, p 617
20. Persson L, Hillered L (1992) Chemical monitoring of neurosurgical intensive care patients using intracerebral microdialysis. J Neurosurg 76: 72–80
21. Pulsinelli WA, Levy DE, Duffy TE (1982) Regional cerebral blood flow and metabolism following transient forebrain ischemia. Ann Neurol 11: 499–509
22. Scheyer RD, During MJ, Spencer DD, Cramer JA, Mattson RH (1994) Measurement of carbamazepine and carbamazepine epoxide in the human brain using in-vivo microdiaysis. Neurology 44: 1469–1472
23. Shuaib A, Ijaz S, Kalra J, Code W (1992) During repetitive forebrain ischemia, postischemic hypothermia protects neurons from damage. Can J Neurol Sci 19: 428–432

24. Siesjö BK (1992) Pathophysiology and treatment of focal cerebral ischemia. Part I: pathophysiology. J Neurosurg 77: 169–184

25. Siesjö BK (1992) Pathophysiology and treatment of focal cerebral ischemia. Part II: mechanisms of damage and treatment. J Neurosurg 77: 337–354

26. Sims NR (1992) Energy metabolism and selective neuronal vulnerability following global cerebral ischemia. Neurochem Res 17: 923–931

27. Sutherland GR, Lesiuk H, Hazendonk P, Peeling J, Buist R, Kozlowski P, Jazinski A, Saunders JK (1992) Magnetic resonance imaging and P31 magnetic resonance spectroscopy study of the effect of temperature on ischemic brain injury. Can J Neurol Sci 19: 317–325

28. Tossman U, Ungerstedt U (1986) Microdialysis in the study of extracellular levels of amino acids in the rat brain. Acta Phys Scand 128: 9–14

29. White BC, Grossman LI, Krause GS (1993) Brain injury by global ischemia and reperfusion: a theoretical perspective on membrane damage and repair. Neurology 43: 1656–1665

Correspondence: Ashfaq Shuaib, M.D., FRCPC, Department of Medicine, Royal University Hospital, Saskatoon, SK, Canada S7N OXO.

Acta Neurochir (1996) [Suppl] 67: 59–62
© Springer-Verlag 1996

Antiepileptic Drug Pharmacokinetics in Patients with Epilepsy Using a New Microdialysis Probe: Preliminary Observations

P.N. Patsalos, M.T. O'Connell, H.C. Doheny, J.W.A.S. Sander, and **S.D. Shorvon**

The National Society for Epilepsy, Chalfont Centre for Epilepsy, Chalfont St Peter, Bucks and Institute of Neurology, The National Hospital for Neurology and Neurosurgery, Queen Square, London, U.K.

Summary

Using a newly developed microdialysis probe which allows continuous monitoring of drugs in blood, we have studied the pharmacokinetics of various antiepileptic drugs (carbamazepine, and its primary metabolite carbamazepine-epoxide, phenytoin, primidone and phenobarbitone) in 5 patients (2 male, 3 female, aged 40–50 years) with intractable epilepsy. It was observed that microdialysate pharmacokinetic profiles were comparable to those obtained by direct blood sampling. Furthermore, patients found the microdialysis probe highly acceptable and desirable and indeed preferable to that of blood sampling

Keywords: Microdialysis probe; blood pharmacokinetics; epilepsy; antiepileptic drugs.

Introduction

Epilepsy affects approximately 1% of the world population at any one time (about 50 million people worldwide) and is the most common serious neurological condition. Because of the long term nature of epilepsy treatment and the unique characteristics and pharmacokinetics of antiepileptic drugs, therapeutic drug monitoring has become invaluable in optimising treatment. The major treatment goal in epilepsy is to stop seizures or to minimise their frequency and also to have minimal concurrent undesirable side-effects. To this end pharmacokinetic considerations are invaluable. Additionally, there is presently a major interest in the development of new more efficacious and less toxic antiepileptic drugs and drugs with improved pharmacokinetic characteristics are of particular interest [1].

Classically, drug pharmacokinetics are undertaken by serial blood sampling using an indwelling catheter. Recently, however, microdialysis, which has contrib-

uted significantly to our understanding of brain neurochemistry, has been applied in studies of blood drug pharmacokinetics in the rat [2] and dog [3]. Sampling of blood by microdialysis has numerous advantages, since it allows continuous monitoring of analytes of interest over an extended period of time and with high temporal resolution. Additional advantages over more traditional blood sampling techniques include: 1. No blood sampling occurs and thus there is no net fluid (blood) loss; 2. No need for constant flushing of catheter to maintain patency and thus no fluid gain; 3. The use of heparin, which can affect drug pharmacokinetics, to maintain catheter patency, is unnecessary; 4. Monitoring of the "free" pharmacologically active fraction is achieved; 5. Enzymes and proteins are excluded from microdialysate and thus post-sampling degradation of the analytes is diminished; 6. Sample preparation prior to analysis can be greatly simplified.

Recently we have developed a miniature, flexible and robust microdialysis probe with specific design features for placing into arteries/veins of patients which can be introduced using standard clinical procedures. Thus for the first time the application of microdialysis in studies of blood pharmacokinetics in man has become feasible. The probe is presently undergoing extensive clinical evaluation and its first use in man in studies of blood levodopa pharmacokinetics in patients with Parkinson's disease has been reported [4]. The present report relates to the current on-going evaluation of the probe in pharmacokinetic studies of antiepileptic drugs in patients with chronic intractable epilepsy. The major features of the evaluation include tolerability, acceptability, and longevity of the probe and pharmacokinetic correlation with that of direct blood sampling.

Methods and Materials

This study was approved by the Joint Ethical Committee of the National Hospital for Neurology and Neurosurgery (Queen Square, London), and all patients gave their consent to be studied. Microdialysis probes were constructed of tubular dialysis membrane (molecule cut-off = 10,000 Daltons) and were sterilised using routine procedures.

To date five patients (2 male, 3 female) with chronic intractable epilepsy resident at the Chalfont Centre for Epilepsy have been studied. Their clinical details are shown in Table 1. They were aged 40–50 years and had no systemic, psychiatric or progressive neurological conditions. All patients were on antiepileptic drug duotherapy, five patients were taking carbamazepine.

After an overnight fast, a microdialysis probe was inserted into a vein of one arm and an 18 gauge Venflon® cannula into a vein of the other arm. The probe was perfused with isotonic saline (0.9% NaCl) at 3 μl/min, using a Harvard perfusion pump (model 22), for the duration of the procedure. After a 30 minute equilibration period for the microdialysis probe, and following a baseline blood sample, patients received their normal morning medication (0800–0900 h). Microdialysate was sampled at 5 minute intervals for 120 minutes and at 10 minute intervals subsequently. Blood was sampled at 15 minute intervals for 60 minutes and at 30 minutes subsequently.

Isotonic saline (0.9% NaCl) was used to flush the Venflon® cannula to maintain patency after withdrawal of each blood sample. Blood samples (10 ml) were collected into tubes containing lithium heparin. Plasma were separated from whole blood by centrifugation in a refrigerated centrifuge at 4°C and stored in microcentrifuge tubes at −70°C until analysis for antiepileptic drug content. At the termination of the procedure the microdialysis probe and Venflon® cannula were removed and their sites of implantation examined for signs of irritation.

All samples (plasma and microdialysates) were analysed within 3 weeks of collection. Carbamazepine, and its primary pharmacologically active metabolite carbamazepine-epoxide, phenytoin, primidone and its primary pharmacologically active metabolite phenobarbitone were measured by high performance liquid chromatography (HPLC) with ultraviolet detection [5]. The HPLC system comprised a Gilson 305 model pump, a rheodyne 7125 fitted with a 20 μl loop and a Kratos Spectroflow 783 UV detector. Microdialysate samples were directly injected into the system. Plasma samples were prepared for analysis of antiepileptic drug total concentrations by deproteination and involved adding 100 μl of acetonitrile to 50 μl of plasma, mixing for 2 minutes and centrifuging for 1 minute. The supernatant extract was then transfered to a clean extraction tube, mixed with 100 μl of HPLC grade water and 10 μl injected into the HPLC system. The procedure used for the determination of the plasma free (non-protein-bound) antiepileptic drug concentrations was essentially the same as for total concentrations, except that samples were first filtered through an Amicon Centrefree Micropartition System (Amicon, Stonehouse, UK) at a temperature of 25°C using a Sorvall RC-5B refrigerated centrifuge (Du Pont, Stevenage, UK). Ten μl of plasma ultrafiltrate were then injected into the HPLC system.

Results

Probe placement was for 370–490 minutes and dialysate sampling periods for the 5 patients (Table 1) were 450, 340, 340, 460 and 420 min respectively. Tolerability and patient acceptability of the new microdialysis probe was excellent. During the entire

Table 1. *Patient Clinical Details*

Patient	Age	Sex	AED medication (mg/day)
1	44	F	CBZ-SR (1600), CLB (10)
2	41	F	PRM (700), CLB (10)
3	46	M	CBZ-SR (1200), SVP (1000)
4	40	M	CBZ-SR (1200), PHT (325)
5	50	F	CBZ-SR (1200), SVP (2000)

CBZ-SR carbamazepine slow release; *CLB* clobazam; *PHT* phenytoin; *PRM* primidone; *SVP* sodium valproate.

study no patient complained of discomfort and no irritation or local inflammatory response was observed at the site of implantation.

Figure 1 shows the plasma concentration versus time profiles for total and free (non-protein-bound) carbamazepine and carbamazepine-epoxide for Patient 4. Figure 2 shows the concurrent profiles for phenytoin. The calculated plasma free fraction (free/total concentration) for each antiepileptic drug studied for the 5 patients is shown in Table 2.

Figure 3 shows the concentration versus time profiles for dialysate carbamazepine and carbamazepine-epoxide compared to that of plasma free concentra-

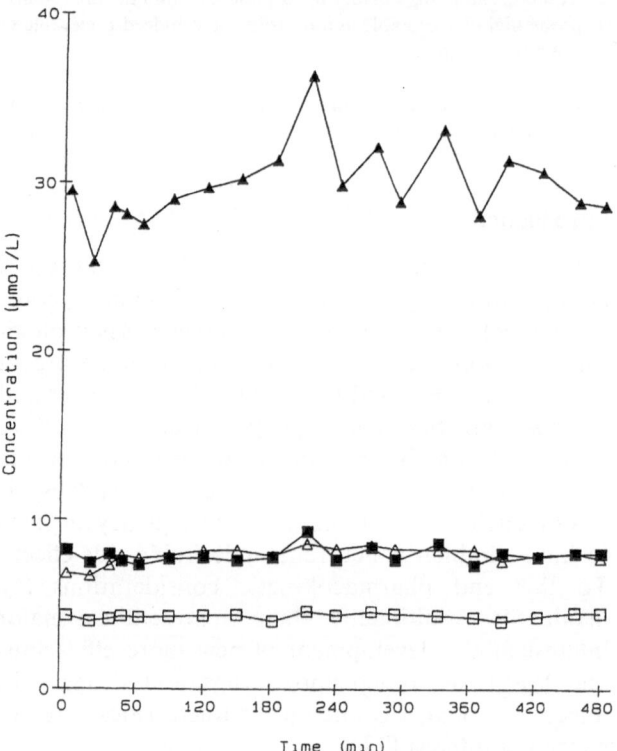

Fig. 1. Concentration versus time profiles for plasma total carbamazepine (▲) and carbamazepine-epoxide (■) and free-non-protein bound carbamazepine (△) and carbamazepine-epoxide (□) in patient 4

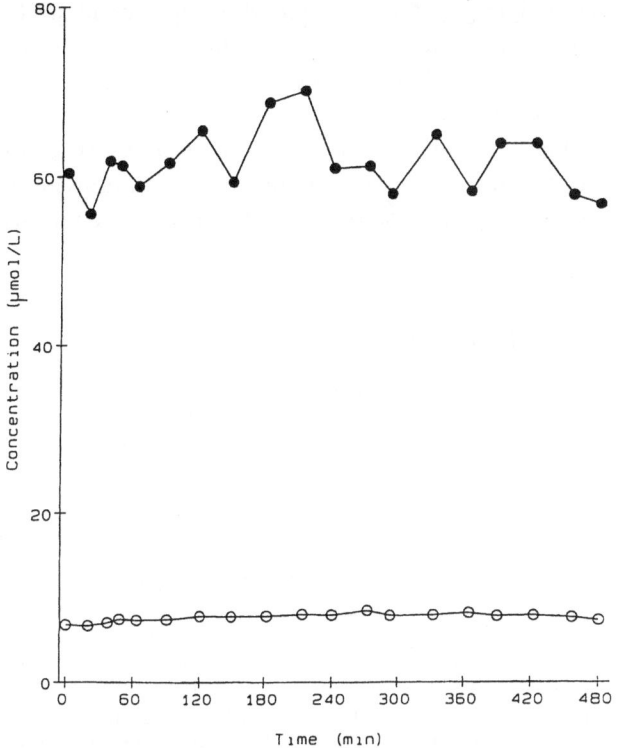

Fig. 2. Concentration versus time profiles for plasma total (●) and free-non-protein bound (○) phenytoin in patient 4

Table 2. *Antiepileptic Drug Plasma Free Fractions*

Patient	1	2	3	4	5
CBZ	0.25		0.20	0.26	0.36
	±0.02		±0.04	±0.02	±0.04
CBZ-E	0.53		0.46	0.54	0.67
	±0.06		±0.06	±0.03	±0.08
PRM		0.34			
		±0.09			
PB		0.64			
		±0.11			
PHT				0.12	
				±0.01	

CBZ carbamazepine; *CBZ-E* carbamazepine-epoxide; *PHT* phenytoin; *PRM* primidone; *PB* phenobarbitone.

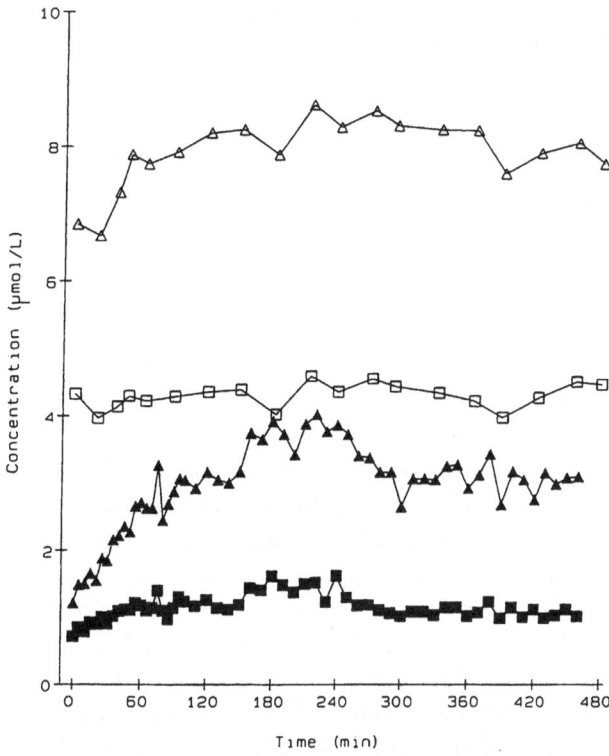

Fig. 3. Comparison of concentration versus time profiles for plasma free-non-protein bound carbamazepine (△) and carbamazepine-epoxide (□) with that of microdialysate carbamazepine (▲) and carbamazepine-epoxide (■) in patient 4

tions of carbamazepine and carbamazepine-epoxide for Patient 4. Dialysate phenytoin and free phenytoin versus time profiles are compared in Fig. 4.

The in vivo recovery of each probe for each antiepileptic drug was determined by comparing microdialysate concentrations with that of free concentrations measured in plasma (Table 3). For carbamazepine and carbamazepine-epoxide, probe recovery was remarkably constant, and were (mean ±sd) 35.5±2.9 and 26.0±0.8, respectively.

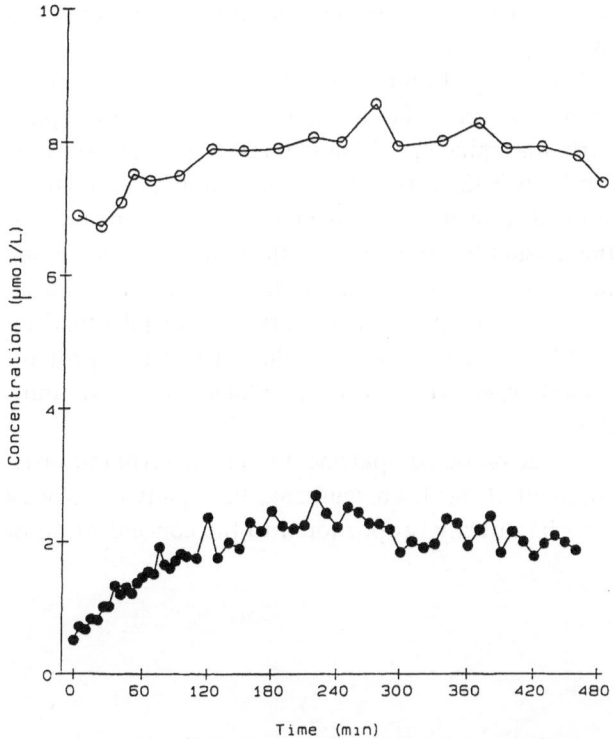

Fig. 4. Comparison of concentration versus time profiles for plasma free-non-protein bound phenytoin (○) with that of microdialysate phenytoin (●) in patient 4

Table 3. *Probe Recovery (%) of the Different Antiepileptic Drugs and Metabolites Compared to Blood Sampling*

	Percentage recovery (%)			
CBZ:	39	32	35	36
CBZ-E:	27	25	26	26
PB	20			
PHT	24			
PRM	100			

Abbreviations see Table 2.

Discussion

This is the first report on the use of microdialysis in studies of blood antiepileptic drug pharmacokinetics in man. Such application has only become feasible as a result of the development, by our group, of a new flexible and robust microdialysis probe. The 5 patients in the present series found the microdialysis probe highly acceptable and indeed preferable to that of blood sampling which confirms previous patient experience of the probe [4]. Although microdialysate sampling occurred over a period of 340 to 460 minutes, the timing is a reflection of inter-dose monitoring of steady state antiepileptic drugs in patients on chronic therapy, and is not a reflection of probe longevity. Thus, microdialysate sampling for longer periods is indeed possible.

From Figs. 1 and 2 it can be seen that there is little inter-dose variability in total and free carbamazepine, carbamazepine-epoxide and phenytoin concentrations (and this is the case with the other antiepileptic drugs studied) as measured from blood sampling. In addition the plasma free fractions for the different antiepileptic drugs (Table 2) are similar to those previously reported [6, 7]. Furthermore microdialysate antiepileptic drug profiles are comparable to that of free non-protein-bound profiles (Figs. 3 and 4) obtained by blood sampling.

As the blood compartment is a hydrodynamic environment, it has been suggested that analyte recovery may be directly proportional to the concentration of the analyte [7]. The probe used in the present study, with its large surface area to maximise analyte recovery, exhibited highly reproducible and acceptable inter-patient recoveries.

Finally, because of the probe's ease of insertion, its maintenance-free characteristics and continuous automated sampling, doctors considered its use clinically desirable.

Acknowledgements

We wish to thank all the enthusiastic patients that agreed to participate in this study and to the nursing staff for their invaluable support.

References

1. Patsalos PN, Sander JWAS (1994) Newer antiepileptic drugs. Towards an improved risk-benefit ratio. Drug Safety 11: 37–67
2. Ståhle L, Segersvärd S, Ungerstedt U (1991) Drug distribution studies with microdialysis. II. Caffeine and theophylline in blood, brain and other tissues in rats. Life Sci 49: 1843–1852
3. Deleu D, Sarre S, Michotte Y, Ebinger G (1994) Simultaneous in vivo microdialysis in plasma and skeletal muscle: a study of the pharmacokinetic properties of levodopa by noncompartmental analysis. J Pharmac Sci 83: 25–28
4. O'Connell MT, Tison F, Quinn NP, Patsalos PN (1994) A newly developed microdialysis probe for monitoring substances in blood of man: Pharmacokinetics of levodopa and its primary metabolite, 3-O-methyldopa in patients with Parkinson's disease: preliminary findings. In: Loulot A *et al* (eds) Monitoring molecules in neuroscience. Publi Typ, Grodignan, pp 53–54
5. Elyas AA, Ratnaraj N, Goldberg VD, Lascelles PT (1982) Routine monitoring of carbamazepine and carbamazepine-10, 11-epoxide in plasma by high performance liquid chromatography using 10-methoxycarbamazepine as internal standard. J Chromatogr 231: 93–101.
6. Levy RH, Schmidt D (1985) Utility of free level monitoring of antiepileptic drugs. Epilepsia 26: 199–205
7. Elyas AA, Patsalos PN, Agbato OA, Brett EM, Lascelles PT (1986) Factors influencing simultaneous concentrations of total and free carbamazepine and carbamazepine-10,11-epoxide in serum of children with epilepsy. Ther Drug Monit 8: 288–292
8. Stenken JA, Topp EM, Southard MZ, Lunte CE (1993) Examination of microdialysis sampling in a well-characterized hydrodynamic system. Anal Chem 65: 2324–2328

Correspondence: P. N. Patsalos, M.D., Pharmacology and Therapeutics Unit, Chalfont Centre for Epilepsy, Chalfont St. Peter, Gerrards Cross, Bucks., SL9 0RJ, U.K.

Acta Neurochir (1996) [Suppl] 67: 63–65
© Springer-Verlag 1996

A New Screwing Device for Fixing a Microdialysis Probe in Critical Care Patients

A. Kanner[1], **A. Mendelowitsch**[1], **H. Langemann**[2], **B. Alessandri**[2], and **O. Gratzl**[1]

[1]University Neurosurgical Clinic and [2] Neurosurgical Laboratory, Department of Research, Kantonsspital, Basel, Switzerland

Summary

We describe a new, easy method which extends the use of clinical microdialysis to neurotrauma patients who primarily do not need a decompressing surgical intervention. In all head trauma patients in whom a Camino ICP-monitor is indicated a second hole (2 mm in diameter) is made, and the MD probe is fixed using the new screwing device. Before clinical use the system was tested during postmortem, confirming correct cortical placement of the probe in almost all cases. Two case reports are presented including their metabolic values. An extension to patients with non-traumatic brain disorders might be a future aspect.

Keywords: Microdialysis; head trauma; critical care; apparatus.

Introduction

Monitoring of metabolic parameters in the extracellular fluid (ECF) of human brain tissue using microdialysis is becoming a more common procedure in critical care patients after head trauma. Ischemia-associated substances have been identified in animal models [1, 2, 4], as well as in human brain dialysates (glucose, lactate, antioxidants, amino acids) [4, 5, 7]. We also developed an on-line pH measurement method [6] enabling real time information from the patients' ECF to be obtained together with the present off-line parameters (glucose, lactate, uric acid, and antioxidants). Microdialysis (MD) as a sampling method for these metabolites has been used in some medical centres during neurosurgical procedures [8, 9] and in neurotrauma patients during their critical care period [7, 10]. Additionally to intracranial pressure (ICP), cerebral perfusion pressure (CPP), routine blood tests and clinical presentation (GCS), MD provides information about the local intracerebral metabolic state. When we started to use neurometabolic monitoring in our critical care patients in 1992, we inserted the microdialysis probe into the cortex. It was either implanted in the operating room through a burr hole, after placing the (Geltec) intracranial-pressure monitor or, in case of craniotomy, at the end of the operation. Thus at this time the use of microdialysis was limited to patients in whom a craniotomy or a burr hole for inserting an ICP-monitor was necessary after a head trauma. After 1993 the Geltec-ICP-monitor was replaced by the Camino-monitoring system in most patients, and neurometabolic monitoring became possible only in patients with craniotomy. Because of this limitation we started the development of a screwing device in order to extend the use of microdialysis to all head trauma patients during their critical care period.

Methods and Material

Inspired by the Camino-ICP screw we created our first prototypes in which a MD probe (CMA 20, 4mm membrane) could be fixed without compressing the tubing or damaging the membrane. In a next step the prototypes were tested 10 times during autopsies. A hole (2 mm diameter) was made in the skull using a hand drill in the frontal region. The screw (Fig. 1) was inserted and a channel for the probe was pre-formed with a special perforator (Fig. 2) to minimize accidental damage. The probe was implanted and fixed by the compression cap. The position of the probe was verified by dye infusion through the probe and subsequent careful histological examination of the relevant cortical region. The final version of the screw (steel and teflon) and its associated instruments (steel) is shown in Figs. 1 and 2. In 1995 we started to use this new system in all our neurotrauma patients in whom an ICP monitoring (Camino ICP monitoring system) was indicated. The whole system including the probe (CMA 20 probes with 4 or 10 mm membrane) was sterilized. The probe was perfused with sterile 0.9% saline at a flow rate of $2\,\mu l/min$, and samples were collected half-hourly. On-line pH and off-line glucose, lactate, uric acid and ascorbic acid were measured, using high pressure liquid chromatography or enzymatic methods. There were no complications such as haemorrhage or infection in these two patients.

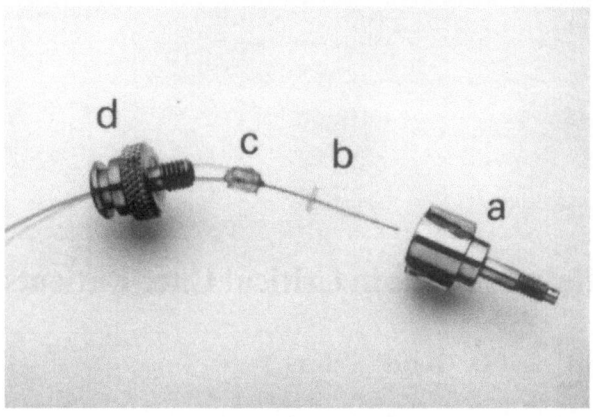

Fig. 1. Screwing device showing *a* screw, *b* silicon sealing ring, *c* microdialysis probe (wings cut off), *d* compression cap

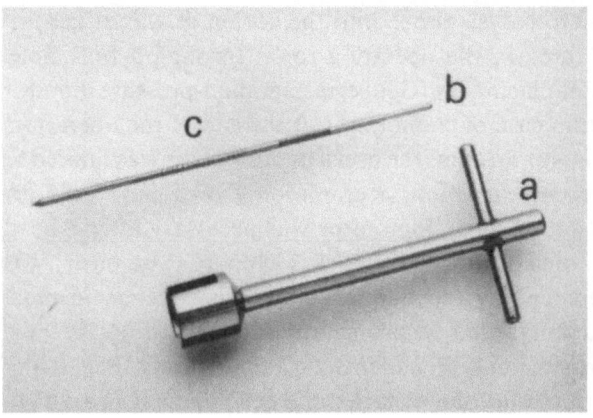

Fig. 2. *a* Screw driver for inserting of the microdialysis screw through the skull and *b* perforator with *c* mm scale for pre-forming a precise channel for the probe

Case Reports

A.L. 22y female (patient 1): High speed motor vehicle accident resulting in a severe closed head injury. At the scene GCS 5, the patient was intubated and transfered to our clinic about 90 min. after the accident. The CT of the neurocranium revealed heavy cerebral oedema and a hypodense right hemisphere. In the emergency room a Camino ICP monitor and a MD screw for neurometabolic monitoring were inserted in the right frontal region (at about 2 cm distance to each other). The initial ICP was over 60 mmHg and the patient was moved to the intensive care unit for acute therapy, resulting in lowering the ICP to normal values and normal CPP (Fig. 3), already within the first hour. However the pH in the dialysate decreased steadily during the first 2.5 days, while all clinical parameters (GCS, ICP, MAP, CPP etc.) remained stable. A cerebral angiogram showed a torsion injury of the right

carotid artery. On day 4 the patient deteriorated clinically (decrease in GCS), with no change in ICP or CPP. On the fifth day, barbiturate coma was induced with no clinical effect. Glucose in the dialysate, which had dropped to zero, started to increase a little after starting nembutal therapy (see Fig. 3). On day 7 a sudden ICP increase to over 90 mmHg occurred, which did not respond to therapy. The patient died a few days later.

J.G. 16y male (patient 2): mountain bike accident resulting in a moderate head injury. At the scene GSC 7, the patient was intubated and transfered to our clinic. The CT revealed cerebral oedema and a slight haemorrhage in the left lateral ventricle. High glucose values in the dialysate throughout the monitoring period, corresponding with good clinical course. Good recovery as the GCS increased up to 9 within the next 10 h. The patient was extubated the next day. The ICP-monitor and the MD probe were removed and the patient was transfered to the ward (GCS 12). GOS good.

Results

Results from the post mortem tests showed that the microdialysis probe was generally wholly or partially in the cortex. Afterwards the screw was used in head trauma patients who required a continuous ICP-monitoring but no other neurosurgical intervention. In our two comatose patients monitoring started about 2.5 hours posttrauma. The time courses of glucose and lactate measurements for both patients are shown in Figs. 3 and 4.

Discussion

The use of microdialysis for neurometabolic monitoring in head trauma patients during their critical care period provides additional information, which in the near future could influence our understanding of secondary brain damage as well as its therapy. With our new screwing device neurometabolic monitoring becomes possible in more head trauma patients. The early and simple implantation makes data available at an early stage after head trauma. No major operation is necessary. The disadvantage is that the exact intracranial position of the probe is unknown. However, as demonstrated during autopsies, the membrane was at least partially located in the cortex in most cases. Findings in patients in whom we used the screw are comparable to those made previously through a burr hole or craniotomy [7, 10]. Making one larger burr hole instead of two smaller ones would be technically

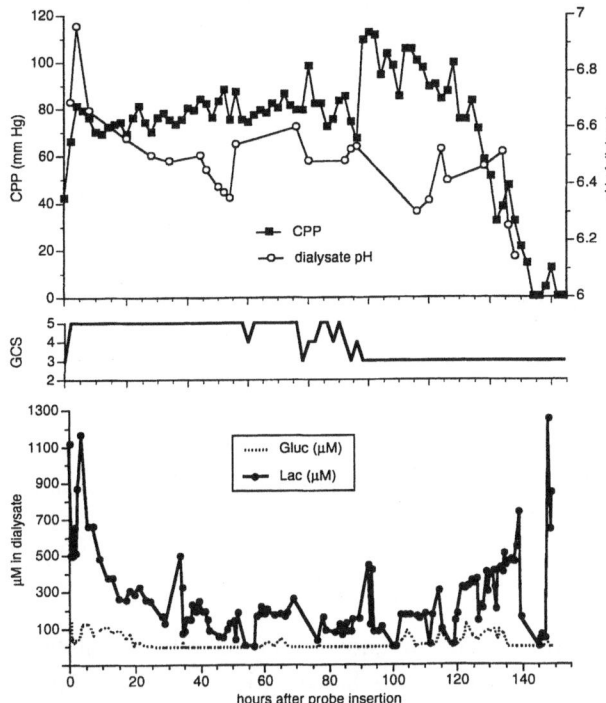

Fig. 3. Time course of clinical and neurometabolic parameters in pat.1. Start of nembutal treatment at 96 h

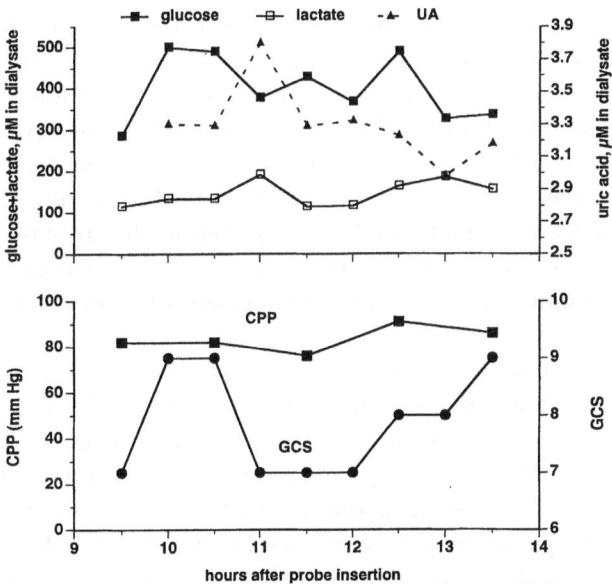

Fig. 4. Time course of clinical and neurometabolic parameters in pat. 2

more complicated, without any additional benefit. A larger diameter means an extended operation and possible interference of the ICP sensor with the micro-diaylsis probe. A recent publication [12] shows that there is a demand for more information about the complex intracerebral biomechanisms taking place

after severe head trauma, parallel to the continuous ICP-monitoring. Through a second hole a sensor was placed on the cortex to measure the regional cerebral blood flow. In the future, we plan routine monitoring, especially long-term measurements using this screwing device. An extension to patients with other cerebral disorders (brain tumor therapy, seizure disorders) might be possible [3, 11].

Acknowledgement

We thank the engineering workshop of the Kantonsspital for their cooperation.

References

1. Benveniste H, Drejer J, Schousboe A, Diemer NH (1984) Elevation of the concentrations of glutamate and aspartate in rat hippocampus during transient cerebral ischemia monitored by microdialysis. J Neurochem 43: 1369–1374
2. Benveniste H and Hüttenmeier PC (1990) Microdialysis—theory and application. Prog Neurobiol 35: 195–215
3. During MJ, Fried I, Leone P, Katz A, Spencer DD (1994) Direct measurement of extracellular lactate in the human hippocampus during spontaneous seizures. J Neurochem 62: 2356–2361
4. Hillered L and Persson L (1991) Microdialysis for metabolic monitoring in cerebral ischemia and trauma; experimental and clinical studies. In: Robinson TE, Justice JB Jr (eds) Microdialysis in the neurosciences. Elsevier, Amsterdam, pp 389–405
5. Hillered L, Persson L, Ponten U, Ungerstedt U (1989) Chemical changes in the extracellular fluid of human cerebral cortex during ischemia measured by intracerebral microdialysis. J Neurochem 52: S 55 B
6. Landolt H, Langemann H, Gratzl O (1993) On-line monitoring of cerebral pH by microdialysis. Neurosurgery 32 (6): 1000–1004
7. Langemann H, Mendelowitsch A, Alessandri B, Landolt H, Gratzl O (1995) Experimental and clinical monitoring of glucose by microdialysis. Clin Neurol Neurosurg 97: 149–155
8. Mendelowitsch A, Langemann H, Landolt H, Gratzl O (1994) Microdialytic monitoring of ischemic changes during brain retraction for aneurysm surgery. In: Nagai H et al (eds) Intracranial pressure IX. Springer, Berlin Heidelberg New York Tokyo, pp 260–263
9. Nilsson OG, Säveland H, Brandt L, Boris-Möller F, Wieloch T (1994) Intracerebral microdialysis of excitatory amino acids in the medial temporal and subfrontal cortex after subarachnoidal hemorrage. In: Louilot A, Durkin T et al (eds) 6th International Conference on in vivo Methods, Seignosse. France Publi Typ, Gradignan, France pp 380–381
10. Persson L, Hillered L (1992) Chemical monitoring of neurosurgical intensive care patients using intracerebral microdialysis. J Neurosurg 76: 72–80
11. Ronquist G, Hugosson R, Sjölander U, Ungerstedt U (1992) Treatment of malignant glioma by a new therapeutic principle. Acta Neurochir (Wien) 114: 8–11
12. Sioutos PJ, Orozco JA, Carter LP, Weinand ME, Hamilton AJ, Williams FC (1995) Continuous regional cerebral cortical blood flow monitoring in head-injured patients. Neurosurgery 36 (5): 943–950

Correspondence: Andrew A. Kanner, M.D., University Neurosurgical Clinic, Kantonsspital, CH-4031 Basel, Switzerland.

Acta Neurochir (1996) [Suppl] 67: 66–69
© Springer-Verlag 1996

A Novel Microdialysis Probe Designed for Clinical Use: Potential Analytical and Therapeutic Applications

J.C. Lehmann[1], **T.R. Jones**[1], **P.K. Mishra**[2], **S. Hamelin**[1], and **S.N. Nair**[1]

[1]Department of Neurosurgery, Medical College of Pennsylvania and Hahnemann University, Philadelphia, PA and [2]College of Medicine, University of Illinois, Peoria, Ill, U.S.A.

Summary

Significant obstacles to the use of microdialysis in the clinic for diagnostic or therapeutic purposes include the production of a dedicated entry port through the skull and the formation of a tract by the insertion of a probe into the parenchyma. We have developed a microdialysis probe that is minimally invasive and can be combined with an intracranial pressure probe, recording electrode, or other intracranial probe, that is minimally invasive. Yet the surface area of this probe is very high, permitting high recovery efficiencies even at relatively high flow rates.

This probe design makes possible minimally invasive measurement of the peroxidation product, uric acid, and excitatory amino acids, two analytes that increase in experimental traumatic brain injury in animals. Moreover, its large surface area makes therapeutic applications of microdialysis probes in the brain potentially feasible. A pilot evaluation of the ability of microdialysis to have therapeutic benefit in limiting experimental excitotoxin lesions induced in rat striatum by N-methyl-D-aspartate (NMDA) is reported.

Keywords: Microdialysis; NMDA; excitotoxicity; stroke; traumatic brain injury.

Introduction

Microdialysis has been used experimentally in animals extensively since the introduction of the technique by Ungerstedt and co-workers [18]. The method has largely replaced those used in the 1970's and 80's to estimate neurotransmitter turnover [2, 8, 19], in the effort to discover the effects of physiological, pharmacological, and pathological variables on the release of specific neurotransmitters, offering important clues concerning their roles. An even partial listing of significant preclinical and basic findings of major significance for neurobiology is beyond the scope of this report.

Only recently have there been clinical studies using microdialysis, but the usefulness of the technique as a routine clinical diagnostic method in brain still faces several significant challenges [4, 5, 15, 17]. (Again, a review of significant contributions involving human microdialysis is beyond the scope of this report.) One such challenge is the requirement to make a dedicated port and tract for the microdialysis probe. This issue has restricted the use of microdialysis probes in the hands of epileptologists to tissues to be resected. Although one may debate the degree of risk of clinically significant damage likely to be caused by insertion of a microdialysis probe, clearly minimizing the invasiveness holds certain advantages. For this reason we have sought to develop a microdialysis probe for human application that could be integrated in the structure and use of other intraparenchymal devices. In so doing, a number of potentially advantageous features have been identified.

Included in the risk/benefit consideration is the potential advantage to the patient of microdialysis. As suggested originally by Ungerstedt and co-workers [18], microdialysis in the brain may have therapeutic benefit. Dialysis technology has become an important therapeutic device for kidney failure. These hollow fiber dialysis membranes have been adapted specifically for use in microdialysis, and have been used with success in the analysis of neurotransmitters in the brain [12, 14]. We have performed a simple experiment to evaluate the potential therapeutic benefit of microdialysis in a neurochemical lesion model mimicking many of the phenomena occurring in stroke and traumatic brain injury, namely, the administration of the excitotoxin N-methyl-D-aspartate (NMDA) in the striatum of the rat. The striatum is convenient for such a study due to its geometry (almost spherical and well suited for reproducible stereotaxic placements) and convenient quantitation of lesions (by measurement of choline acetyltransferase (ChAT), an enzyme specific to cholinergic interneurons of the striatum [9–11]. Specifically, it was investigated whether continuous microdialysis during 24 hours could reduce the neurotoxicity caused by NMDA in rat striatum.

Materials and Methods

Human Microdialysis Probe Construction

Human microdialysis probes were constructed of polyimide and fused silica tubing (Micropolyx, Chattanooga TN) and Spectrapor 8 kDa methylcellulose dialysis membrane (Spectrum, Houston TX). A large central lumen in the "carrier tubing" (Fig. 1) was provided to allow the passage of a primary probe (ICP, electrode, etc.) with o.d. just small enough to fit inside the dialysis tubing, accepting two fused silica lines as input and output placed at the bottom and the top of the dialysis membrane respectively (see Fig. 1). The lower and upper edges of the dialysis membrane were anchored with cyanoacrylate. The inner diameter of the large tubing (Fig. 1) was selected as

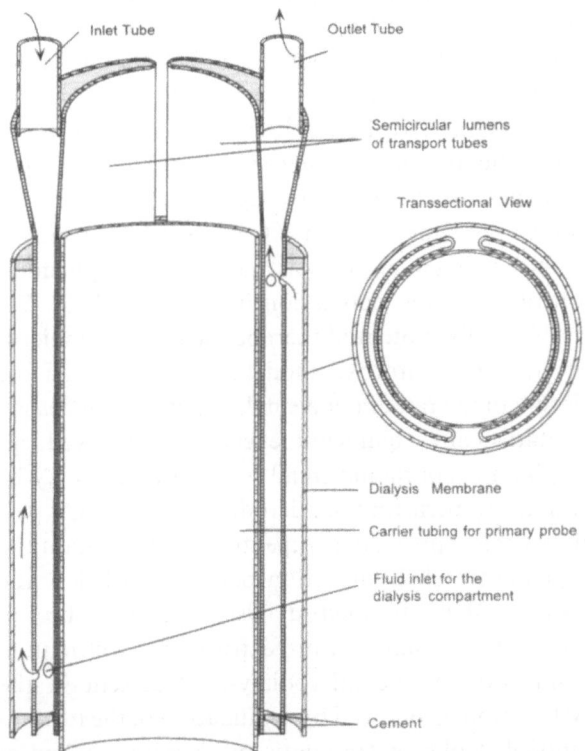

Fig. 1. Human microdialysis probe in cross section. The "carrier tubing" is designed to slide over a "primary probe" (intracranial pressure probe, electrophysiological recording electrode, injection cannula, etc.). Dialysis membrane (8 kDa cut-off) surrounds the carrier tubing, and is cemented to the carrier tubing at its bottom, and at the top. Inlet tubing made of fused silica enters one side and descends to near the bottom of the dialysis membrane. Outlet tubing exits from the opposite side of the probe, near the top of the dialysis membrane

a function of the outer diameter of the primary probe (ICP, electrode, etc.) intended for simultaneous use. The carrier tubing was pierced to allow the input and output lines to travel inside this carrier tubing. The carrier tubing may be sufficiently long to exit the cranial port to allow adjustment of the depth of the active part of the probe along the length of the primary probe.

Model Lesions in Rats

Male Wistar rats (200–240 g) were implanted with guide cannulas (Harvard Instruments, Cambridge MA) anchored with dental acrylic cement and stainless steel screws. Twenty-four hours later, a loop-style microdialysis probe with a fused silica tubing injection port extending 2 mm below the bottom of the 3 mm dialysis loop was inserted, and the freely moving animals placed in a plexiglas cage with the microdialysis loop connected to a liquid swivel (Instech Instruments, Plymouth Meeting PA). One group of animals was perfused at a rate of 8.5 μl/min with artificial CSF for 30 min prior to and 24 hours following injection of the neuroexcitotoxin N-methyl-D-aspartate (NMDA) (100 nmol in 1 μl artificial CSF). A second group of animals underwent identical insertion of the microdialysis probe and NMDA injection but received no perfusion through the microdialysis probe at any time. All animals were sacrificed 7 days after NMDA administration, the striatum dissected at 4°C, and choline acetyltransferase measured by the method of Fonnum [3]. This method has been used extensively to characterize neuroprotectants, in particular NMDA receptor antagonists that have been found effective in blocking neurodegeneration in ischemic stroke models [1].

Results

Human Microdialysis Probe

The prototype human microdialysis probe was tested using the Camino ICP probe as primary probe. The entry port used for this ICP probe accepted the carrier tubing and input/output fused silica tubings without restricting flow. The total active area of the prototype probe (4 mm o.d. × 30 mm length) was 350 mm^2 [2], which may be compared to a surface area approximating 3.8 mm^2 [2] for most microdialysis probes made for use in animals. The increase in effective surface area translates into a greater potential perfusion rate without loss in recovery efficiency of analytes. When tested at 100 μl/min, the probe functioned without failure of any junctions. The probe was tested to pressures as high as 600 mm Hg (approximately three times higher than ICP pressures expected to be encountered). The combination probe has not yet been tested in humans.

Experimental Therapeutic Efficacy in Rat Striatal Excitotoxin Model

Rats receiving 100 nmol NMDA injections demonstrated contralateral circling but no jumping, clonic-tonic convulsions, or other overt signs of neurotoxicity

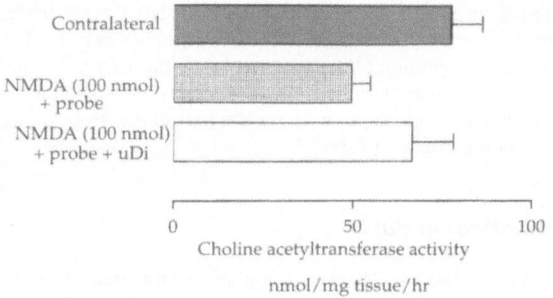

Fig. 2. Effects of microdialysis on excitotoxicity caused by N-methyl-D-aspartate (NMDA). All rats received an implantation of microdialysis probe with injection port 2 mm ventral to the 3 mm microdialysis loop. All animals received an injection of 100 nmol NMDA in 1 µl. Choline acetyltransferase activity is expressed as nmol ACh/mg tissue/h [3]. There were no statistically significant differences between the choline acetyltransferase values of the two groups of contralateral striata, so these values were pooled. The differences between the two groups of striata injected with NMDA was not statistically significant using Student's two-tailed T-test

acutely. There were no behavioral differences noted between rats receiving microdialysis and those rats receiving only microdialysis probes. The results of the radioenzymatic assays to measure the difference between these two groups are given in Fig. 2. Although the magnitude of decrease in ChAT activity was lower in the group receiving microdialysis than the corresponding control group, the difference failed to achieve statistic significance by Student's two-tailed test (although significant by a one-tailed test $P < 0.05$).

Discussion

The two major obstacles to implementation of microdialysis clinically deal with risk and benefit. The work presented here represents preliminary steps to address both of these issues.

The risk associated with clinical microdialysis can be minimized by the simplification of the probe design, and particularly the integration of microdialysis probes with intracranial probes currently in use neurosurgically, avoiding the need to produce a separate twist-drill hole and separate tract. This combination probe permits flexibility of design, including the ability to scale up in size. Increased size has both specific advantages and disadvantages.

Potential advantages include a larger collection surface which may permit decreased depletion of neurotransmitters and other substances in the parenchyma at low flow rates (1–3 µl/min)—an effect that otherwise may create artefactual physiological conditions in the brain [16]. The ability to sample other parameters

of interest, such as intracranial pressure, electrophysiological parameters, etc. enhances the ability to interpret microdialysis data in a meaningful way [13]. Alternatively, the larger collection surface permits the use of higher flow rates, resulting in larger amounts of sample recovered and consequently more analyte, allowing more analytes to be measured with reduced exigence on the analytical sensitivity. Further, very high flow rates may be used to intentionally remove extracellular substances, including neurotoxic substances, such as nitric oxide, platelet aggregating factor, interleukin-1, endothelins, a variety of peroxidative molecules, to name just a few [7], that are present in acute neurodegenerative disorders. Current pharmacological intervention against the plethora of toxins released is impractical at best. Removal of all these toxic agents may offer the best therapeutic approach possible.

With respect to disadvantages, the larger volume of the human probe is likely to reduce the time resolution. A larger probe is likely to affect a larger region of brain, and this may undesirably perturb the system under study from its physiological state.

Ultimately, benefit to the patient will require either advances in real-time or rapid off-line analysis of microdialysate [6], or else the proof of an intrinsic therapeutic benefit of microdialysis. The potential therapeutic benefit, originally suggested by Ungerstedt, has received support from a recent study in which it was shown that microdialysis may reduce the phenomenon of spreading depression in the brain [16]. We have tested the potential therapeutic benefit of microdialysis in the excitotoxin model commonly used in the striatum of the rat, under a single experimental design. No statistically significant effect was observed, although an encouraging trend was noticed. It may be necessary to perform the microdialysis for longer periods of time to provide therapeutic benefit. In addition, the geometry of the injection port (2 mm below the lowest point of the microdialysis loop) may be too demanding a design. Future experiments will require optimization of the microdialysis treatment in the NMDA model, followed by a validation of the method in model stroke or traumatic brain injury, a line of investigation we are currently pursuing.

References

1. Boast CA, Gerhardt SC, Pastor G, Lehmann J, Etienne PE, Liebman JM (1988) The N-methyl-D-aspartate antagonists CGS 19755 and CPP reduce ischemic brain damage in gerbils. Brain Res 442: 345–348

2. Cheney DL, Lehmann J, Cosi C, Wood PL (1989) Determination of acetylcholine dynamics. In: Boulton AB, Baker GB, Juorio AV (eds) Neuromethods, Vol 12. Drugs as tools in neurotransmitter research. Humana, Clifton, NJ, pp 443–495

3. Fonnum F (1975) A rapid radiochemical method for the determination of choline acetyltransferase. J Neurochem 24: 407–409

4. Hillered L, Persson L, Ponten U, Ungerstedt U (1990) Neurometabolic monitoring of the ischaemic human brain using microdialysis. Acta Neurochir (Wien) 102: 91–97

5. Hillered L, Persson L, Ungerstedt U (1990) Chemical changes in the extracellular fluid of human cerebral cortex during ischemica measured by intracerebral microdialysis. J Neurochem 52 [Suppl]: S55B

6. Landolt H, Langemann H, Gratzl O (1993) On-line monitoring of cerebral pH by microdialysis. Neurosurgery 32: 1000–1004

7. Landolt H, Lutz TW, Langemann H, Stauble D, Mendelowitsch A, Gratzl O, Honegger CG (1992) Extracellular antioxidants and amino acids in the cortex of the rat: monitoring by midrodialysis of early ischemic changes. J Cerebral Blood Flow Metab 12: 96–102

8. Langer SZ, Lehmann J (1988) Presynaptic receptors on catecholamine neurones. In: Trendelenburg U, Weiner N (eds) Handbook of experimental pharmacology, Vol 90/I. Springer, Berlin Heidelberg New York Tokyo, pp 419–507

9. Lehmann J, Ferkany JW, Schaeffer P, Coyle JT (1985) Dissociation between the excitatory and "excitotoxic" effects of quinolinic acid analogs on the striatal cholinergic interneuron. J Pharmacol Exp Ther 232: 873–882

10. Lehmann J, Fibiger HC (1979) Acetylcholinesterase and the cholinergic neuron. Life Sci 5: 1161–1174

11. Lehmann J, Schneider J, McPherson S, Murphy DE, Bernard P, Tsai C, Bennett DA, Pastor G, Steel DJ, Boehm C, Cheney DL, Liebman JM, Williams M, Wood PL (1987) CPP, a selective NMDA-type receptor antagonist: characterization in vitro and in vivo. J Pharmacol Exp Ther 240: 737–746

12. Lehmann J, Valentino R, Robine V (1992) Cortical norepinephrine release elicited in situ by N-methyl-D-aspartate (NMDA) receptor stimulation: a microdialysis study. Brain Res 599: 171–174

13. Ludvig N, Mishra PK, Yan Q-S, Lasley SM, Burger RL Jobe PC (1992) The paradoxical effect of NMDA receptor stimulation on electrical activity of the sensorimotor cortex in freely behaving rats: analysis by combined EEG-intracerebral microdialysis. Synapse 12: 87–96

14. Ludvig N, Mishra PK, Yan QS, Lasley SM, Burger RL Jobe PC (1992) The combined EEG-intracerebral microdialysis technique: a new tool for neuropharmacological studies on freely behaving animals. J Neurosci Methods 43: 129–137

15. Meyerson BA, Linderoth B, Karlsson H, Ungerstedt U (1989) Microdialysis in the human brain: extracellular measurements in the thalamus of Parkinsonian patients. Life Sci 46: 301–308

16. Obrenovitch TP, Zilkha E, Urenjak J (1995) Intracerebral microdialysis: electrophysiological evidence of a critical pitfall. J Neurochem 64: 1884–1887

17. Persson L, Hillered L (1992) Chemical monitoring of neurosurgical intensive care patients using intracerebral microdialysis. J Neurosurg 76: 72–80

18. Ungerstedt U (1984) Measurement of neurotransmitter release by intracranial dialysis. Measure of neurotransmit release in vivo pp 81–105

19. Wood PL, Cheney DL (1985) Gas chromatography-mass fragmentography of amino acids. In: Marsden CA (ed) Measurements of neurotransmitter release in vivo. Wiley, NY, pp 51–80

Correspondence: John C. Lehmann, Ph.D., Department of Neurosurgery, Mail Stop 407, Medical College of Pennsylvania and Hahnemann University, Philadelphia PA 19102-1192 U.S.A.

Acta Neurochir (1996) [Suppl] 67: 70–74
© Springer-Verlag 1996

Microdialytic Monitoring During a Cardiovascular Operation

H. Langemann[1], **J. Habicht**[2], **A. Mendelowitsch**[3], **A. Kanner**[3], **B. Alessandri**[1], **H. Landolt**[4], and **O. Gratzl**[3]

[1]Department of Research, [2]Thoracic and Cardiovascular Clinic, [3]Neurosurgical Clinic, Kantonsspital, Basel, and [4]Neurosurgical Clinic, Kantonsspital, Aarau, Switzerland

Summary

In an aorta-coronary bypass operation, the heart is excluded from the circulation for many minutes, leading to ischaemia. During this time the heart is cooled in order to mitigate damage. Microdialysis has been shown to be very suitable for detecting ischaemic changes e.g. in brain. We therefore used this method to study the time courses of several neurochemical parameters which have been shown to indicate ischaemia in animal models (ascorbic acid, glutathione, cysteine, uric acid, glucose, lactate and pH), during such a bypass operation. Three patients were investigated, the microdialysis probe being inserted into the interventricular septum of the heart. Our results show that microdialysis is technically feasible in the human heart in a clinical setting, although the operation becomes more demanding for the surgeon. All the above-mentioned parameters could be detected in the heart muscle. Some of them showed changes characteristic of ischaemia, and the effects of cooling on the metabolism could also be noted. Long term measurements are planned to enable delayed damage to be disclosed.

Keywords: Microdialysis; heart; ischaemia; metabolism.

Introduction

During aorta-coronary bypass operations the heart is excluded from the circulation for many minutes, leading to ischaemia. To attenuate damage, the heart is perfused with cooled cardioplegic solution. Our aim was to see if microdialysis of the heart muscle could be used to study this ischaemia during the course of the operation, i.e. before and after use of the heart-lung machine (HLM), with and without cardioplegia. The technique of microdialysis has been applied by several groups in order to study ischaemia and reperfusion in the heart of the dog or rat; however, cooling was not used in these animal models, in which cardiac ischaemia was produced by ligature of one or more of the coronary arteries. Parameters measured during is-

chaemia included norepinephrine [12], hydroxyl radicals [12, 13], lactate [14] and total adenine nucleotide breakdown products [6], as well as xanthine, inosine, hypoxanthine and uric acid separately [14]. Hamberger *et al.* have used microdialysis to study the time course of changes in amino acids in the myocardium of about 30 postoperative patients over several days (data communicated at the First International Meeting on Clinical Aspects of Microdialysis, Basel, Switzerland, March 1995). They used a specially constructed probe for this purpose [2]. We and other authors have used cerebral microdialysis to find out which parameters show altered levels in the extracellular fluid of the ischaemic zone after middle cerebral artery occlusion in the rat. Such parameters include on-line pH [7], the antioxidants ascorbic acid (Asc) [4], glutathione (GSH) and cysteine (Cys), the putative marker for free radical activity, uric acid (UA) [9], glucose as energy source [10] and lactate as indicator of anaerobic metabolism [3]. We have also applied these parameters to assess ischaemic situations in patients (during neurointensive care and neurovascular operations) [8, 11]. We have therefore used the very same parameters for this preliminary study of cardiac ischaemia and reperfusion.

Methods

Up till now, 3 patients have been investigated. The course of the operation is outlined in Fig. 1. There are 5 phases: in phase 1, the heart is beating normally. In phase 2, the HLM is started, the whole body being slightly cooled (32°C). In phase 3, the heart is excluded from the circulation by clamping the aorta and thus becomes ischaemic; it is cooled by perfusion with cardioplegic solution at 8°C (antegrade cold blood cardioplegia solution). At this point the

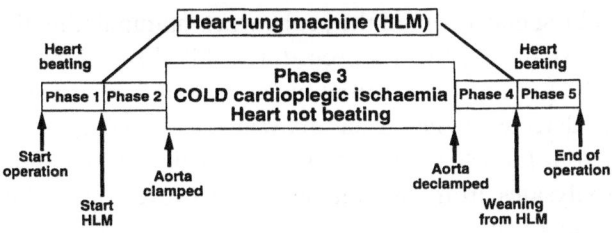

Fig. 1. Diagram showing the course of an aorta-coronary bypass operation

aorta-coronary bypasses are made. In patients 1, 2 and 3, cold ischemia lasted 45, 18 and 41 min and minimal temperatures in the septum were 19.2°, 11.8° and 14.5° respectively. The minimal temperature reached during cold ischaemia is dependent on the condition of the coronary blood vessels before operation. In phase 4 the aorta is declamped; there is warming and reperfusion, leading to the end of ischaemia and the heart is weaned from the HLM. Finally in phase 5 the heart has taken over circulation completely.

The apparatus for the microdialysis (pump and fraction collector) was obtained from CMA Microdialyis, Stockholm, Sweden. A sterile microdialysis probe (CMA 20, 4mm membrane) was implanted into the interventricular septum of the heart 20–55 mins before the HLM was started. To enable implantation, a small hole was made in the myocardium using the temperature probe routinely used during the operation. Probes were perfused with 0.9% saline at 4 µl/min and

samples were collected every 10 mins. The tubing between the probe and the collector had a length of ca 1m, including the on-line pH meter [7], leading to a delay of about 10 min in sample collection. The probes were removed after one or two samples had been collected during phase 5.

The dialysate was analysed as follows: 1) In 5 µl, Asc, UA, Cys and GSH, using high pressure liquid chromatography and electrochemical detection with a gold electrode set at 0.65V [5]; 2) In 15 µl, lactate by a fluorimetric enzymatic method [1]; 3) In 15 µl, glucose, colorimetrically using a kit (Trinder from Sigma); 4) On-line pH [7].

After the end of the operation, the in vitro recovery of the probe used was measured for the relevant parameters at 37° and 0°.

Results

Average values in the dialysates before operation with our microdialysis conditions were: Asc, 2.72 µM; UA, 36.6 µM; GSH, 2.04 µM; glucose, 270 µM; lactate, 167 µM (all n = 3). Values for Cys varied greatly: 2.3 µM, 0.24 µM, and in one case it was not detectable.

The time courses of changes in dialysate concentrations during the operations are shown in Figs. 2, 3, and 4. The time points were adjusted by 10 mins, to allow for the delay in probe collection. During cold is-

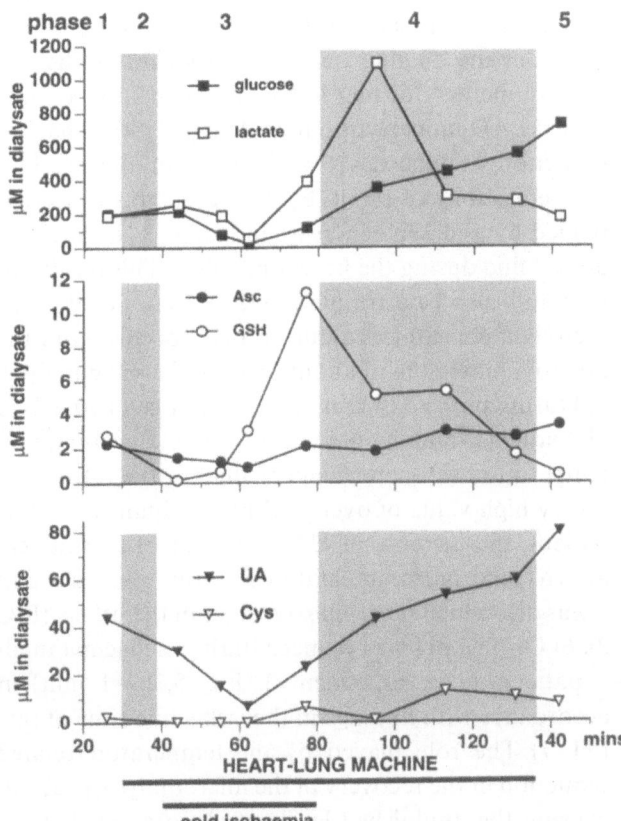

Fig. 2. The time course of levels of neurochemical parameters in human cardiac dialysates during an aorta-coronary bypass operation. Patient 1. For an explanation of the phases, see Fig. 1

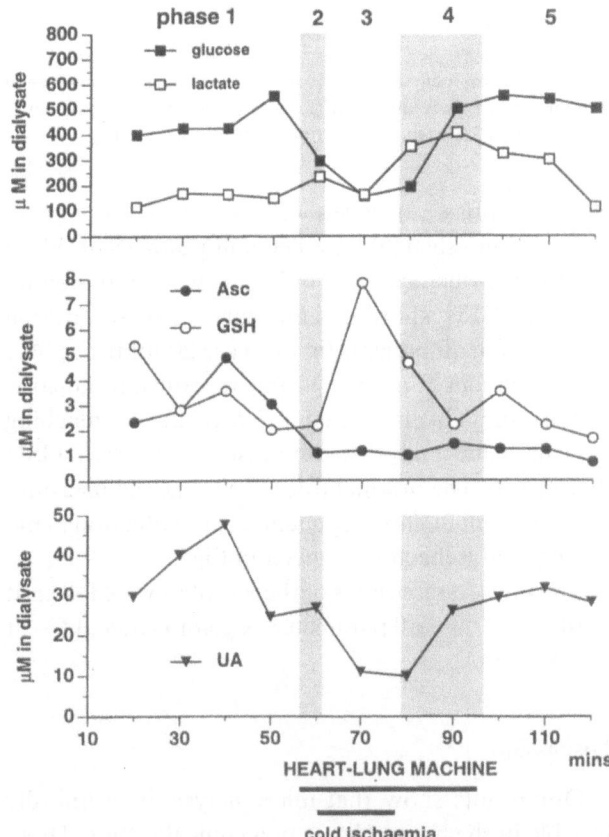

Fig. 3. The time course of levels of neurochemical parameters in human cardiac dialysates during an aorta-coronary bypass operation. Patient 2. For an explanation of the phases, see Fig. 1

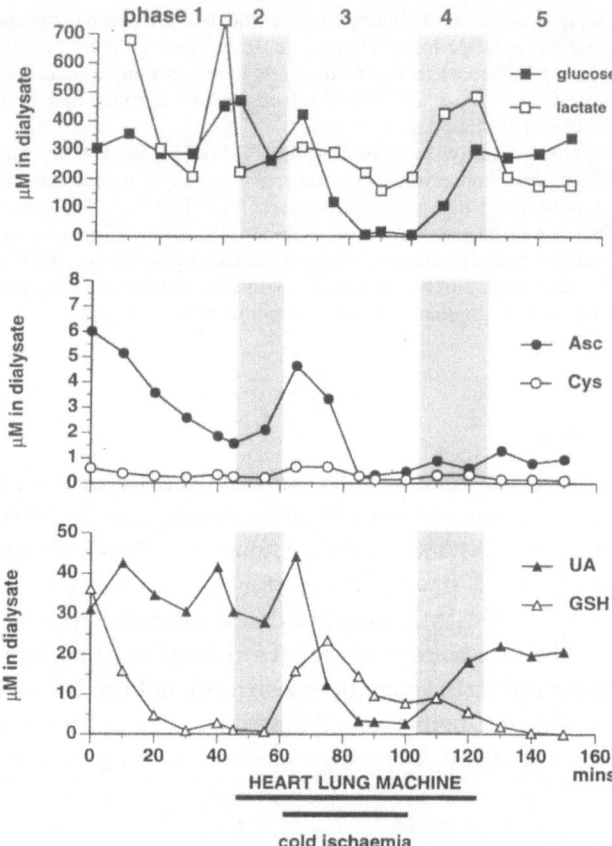

Fig. 4. The time course of levels of neurochemical parameters in human cardiac dialysates during an aorta-coronary bypass operation. Patient 3. For an explanation of the phases, see Fig. 1

chaemia (phase 3), levels of glucose and UA were greatly diminished (glucose becoming unmeasurable in 2 patients), whereas those of lactate were only slightly reduced. GSH showed temporary increases during ischaemia in all patients (in one case 20-fold), and Asc in one patient (Fig. 4). During reperfusion, glucose, lactate and UA increased rapidly, lactate reaching a peak value and then diminishing, whereas GSH diminished. The original trace of on-line pH measurement (Patient 3), showing a temporary reduction in pH during cold ischaemia, is given in Fig. 5.

The in vitro recoveries of the 3 probes were lower at 0° than at 37° for all parameters (e.g. for lactate, 11% at 37°, 5% at 0°).

Discussion

Our results show that microdialysis is technically feasible in the human heart in a clinical setting. However, the operation becomes more demanding for the surgeon because the tubing gets in the way of operational procedures, the probe may be dislocated or the tubing may drop off the probe when manipulating the heart during bypass procedures. All the parameters which we have measured in cerebral dialysates could be detected in the cardiac dialysates. These compounds to our knowledge, have never been measured in microdialysates from human hearts. However, in a dog model using temporary occlusion of the left anterior descending coronary artery (LAD), UA and lactate have been determined in heart dialysates before operation [14]. The UA level (4 µM) was almost 10 times less, whereas lactate (390 µM) was slightly higher than the value which we found in humans before the operation. This might partially be explained by differing microdialysis conditions.

Although we cannot draw many conclusions from these preliminary measurements with only 3 patients, there are some interesting features. 1) Increases in Asc and GSH have also been found during cerebral ischaemia [9]. 2) The reduction of the free radical scavenger GSH during the reperfusion phase is in agreement with the finding of increased OH-radical activity at this stage in an animal model [13]. 3) UA, which increases slowly in the cerebral focal ischaemic zone [9] is markedly reduced during phase 3 (cold ischaemia). This can probably be attributed to the effects of the cooling on the metabolism as there is a small increase during ischaemia in the above-mentioned LAD model without cooling [14]. 4) A marked reduction in glucose is also found in the cerebral ischaemic zone of rats [10]. However, this is accompanied by a massive increase in lactate [4], which we do not find during the heart operation. This result can probably also be attributed to the effect of cooling, as there is a constant rise during LAD occlusion in the dog to a maximum of about 15-fold after 60 min [14]. 5) During phase 4 (warming) there is a lactate peak in all patients, and in patient 1, where the minimum temperature was rather higher than in the other two, a very high value of over 1 mM was obtained. In this patient, the increase in UA (indicator of free radical activity and purine breakdown) during phases 4 and 5 was also much more massive than in the others (Fig. 2). 6) On-line pH was reduced during ischaemia in all 3 patients (e. g. in patient 3, Fig. 5, by 1 unit) in accordance with findings in the ischaemic zone of rats [7]. 7) The role played by the temperature-related reduction in the recovery of the microdialysis probe in causing the diminished levels of glucose and UA remains to be elucidated.

It is known that the effects of ischaemic damage in the heart are often seen only after several hours. In the

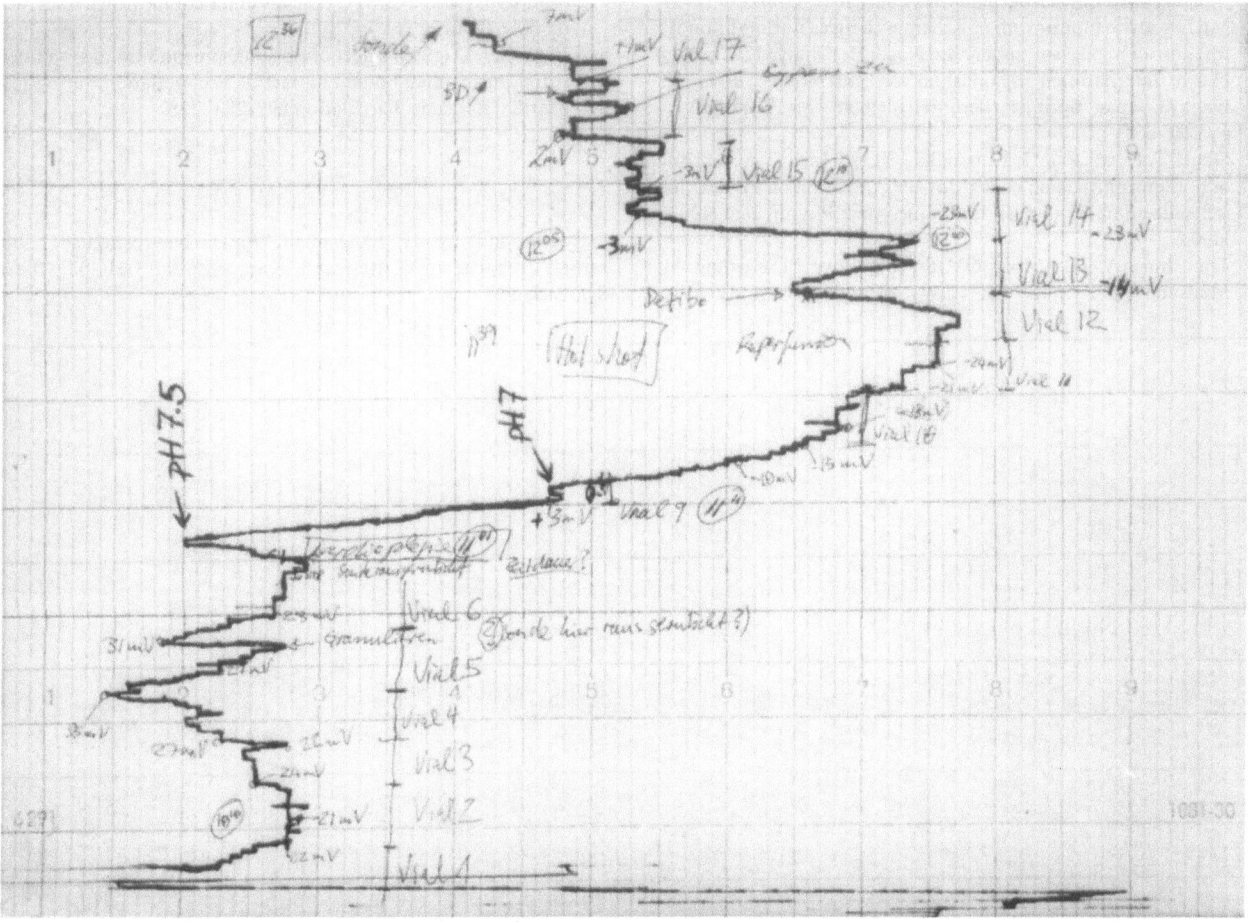

Fig. 5. Original trace showing changes in on.-line pH during an aorta-coronary bypass operation. Patient 3

future we would therefore like to continue microdialysis into the post-operational period, to try to detect this delayed damage.

References

1. Bergmeyer HU (1974) Methoden der Enzymatischen Analyse. Verlag Chemie, Weinheim, pp 1515–1518
2. Hamberger A, Jacobson I, Larsson S, Lönnroth P, Nyström B, Sandberg M (1991) Microdialysis techniques for studying brain amino acids in the extracellular fluid: basic and clinical studies. In: Robertson F, Justice J (eds) Microdialysis in neurosciences. Elsevier, Amsterdam, pp 407–423
3. Hillered L, Hallstrom A, Segersvard S, Persson L, Ungerstedt U (1989) Dynamics of extracellular metabolites in the striatum after middle cerebral artery occlusion in the rat monitored by intracerebral microdialysis [published erratum appears in J Cereb Blood Flow Metab 10(1): 149–151, 1990]. J Cereb Blood Flow Metab 9: 607–616
4. Hillered L, Persson L, Bolander HG, Hallstrom A, Ungerstedt U (1988) Increased extracellular levels of ascorbate in the striatum after middle cerebral artery occlusion in the rat monitored by intracerebral microdialysis. Neurosci Lett 95: 286–290
5. Honegger CG, Langemann H, Krenger W, Kempf A (1989) Liquid chromatographic determination of common water-soluble antioxidants in biological samples. J Chromatogr 487: 463–468
6. Kuzmin AI, Tskitishvili OV, Serebryakova LI, Saprygina TV, Kapelko VI, Medvedev OS (1992) Cardiac microdialysis measurement of extracellular adenine nucleotide breakdown products during regional ischemia and reperfusion in canine heart—protective effect of propranolol against reperfusion injury. J Cardiovasc Pharmacol 20: 961–968
7. Landolt H, Langemann H, Gratzl O (1993) On-line monitoring of cerebral pH by microdialysis. Neurosurgery 32: 1000–1004
8. Landolt H, Langemann H, Mendelowitsch A, Gratzl O (1994) Neurochemical monitoring and on-line pH measurements using brain microdialysis in patients in intensive care. Acta Neurochir (Wien) [Suppl] 60: 475–478
9. Landolt H, Lutz TW, Langemann H, Stauble D, Mendelowitsch A, Gratzl O, Honegger CG (1992) Extracellular antioxidants and amino acids in the cortex of the rat—monitoring by microdialysis of early ischemic changes. J Cereb Blood Flow Metab 12: 96–102
10. Langemann H, Landolt H, Mendelowitsch A, Gratzl O (1994) Experimental and clinical monitoring of glucose by cerebral microdialysis. In: Louilot A, Durkin T et al (eds) 6th International Conference on in vivo methods. Seignosse, France, Publi Typ, Gradignan, France, pp 382–383

11. Mendelowitsch A, Langemann H, Landolt H, Gratzl O (1994) Microdialytic monitoring of ischemic changes during brain retraction for aneurysm surgery. In: Nagai H, Kamiya K *et al* (eds) Ninth International Symposium on Intercranial Pressure, Nagoya, Japan. Springer, Berlin Heidelberg New York Tokyo, pp 260–263

12. Obata T, Hosokawa H, Yamanaka Y (1994) In vivo monitoring of norepinephrine and center-dot-oh generation on myocardial ischemic injury by dialysis technique. Am J Physiol 266: H903–H908

13. Timoshin AA, Tskitishvili OV, Serebryakova LI, Kuzmin AI, Medvedev OS, Ruuge EK (1994) Microdialysis study of ischemia-induced hydroxyl radicals in the canine heart. Experientia 50: 677–679

14. Vanwylen D (1994) Effect of ischemic preconditioning on interstitial purine metabolite and lactate accumulation during myocardial ischemia. Circulation 89: 2283–2289

Correspondence: H. Langemann, Ph.D., Neurosurgical Laboratory, Department of Research, Kantonsspital, CH-4031 Basel, Switzerland.

Index of Keywords

SpringerNews

A. Baethmann, O. S. Kempski,
N. Plesnila, F. Staub (eds.)

Mechanisms of Secondary Brain Damage in Cerebral Ischemia and Trauma

1996. 52 figures. VIII, 122 pages.
Cloth DM 180,–, öS 1260,–, US $ 139.50
Reduced price for subscribers to "Acta Neurochirurgica":
Cloth DM 162,–, öS 1134,–
ISBN 3-211-82817-6
Acta Neurochirurgica, Supplement 66

The publication is a progress report of the understanding of secondary brain damage from head injury and cerebral ischemia. The spectrum reaches from the molecular- and cell biological level up to the complex issues of clinical management. Specific topics on cerebral ischemia are concerned with apoptosis, inflammation, acidosis, cellular Ca^{2+}-overflow, the role of the stimulatory input for maintenance of functional competence in stroke, effects of brain grafting in infarction, and the current state of glutamate antagonization or reestablishment of cerebral blood flow by thrombolysis, among others. Novel data on head injury relate with the cell biological response of the damaged axon, the activation of microglia, the role of β-amyloid precursor protein in the later development of Alzheimer's disease, and the current understanding of neuronal regeneration. Aspects of management and treatment have a spectrum from novel antioxidants to international consensus efforts.

SpringerNeurosurgery

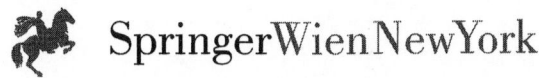 SpringerWienNewYork

P.O.Box 89, A-1201 Wien • New York, NY 10010, 175 Fifth Avenue
Heidelberger Platz 3, D-14197 Berlin • Tokyo 113, 3-13, Hongo 3-chome, Bunkyo-ku

SpringerNews

R. Fahlbusch, W. J. Bock, M. Brock, M. Buchfelder, M. Klinger (eds.)

Modern Neurosurgery of Meningiomas and Pituitary Adenomas

1996. 69 figures. VIII, 112 pages.
Cloth DM 180,–, öS 1260,–, US $ 143.00
Reduced price for subscribers to "Acta Neurochirurgica":
Cloth DM 162,–, öS 1134,–
ISBN 3-211-82779-X
Acta Neurochirurgica, Supplement 65

This book presents todays level of knowledge about pituitary adenomas and meningiomas. Molecular biology has added significant new information to our understanding of these tumors which in turn affects the current treatment of these tumor types. Pituitary adenomas require meticulous study not only in the diagnosis, but also in the analysis of the right kind of therapy which includes surgery, radiosurgery and medical treatment. Great progress has also been achieved in research on the hormonal aspects of meningiomas. Clinical symptomatology and treatment of these tumors depend largely on the localization of these meningiomas. The special problems associated with meningiomas of the cavernous sinus differ greatly from those of ventral foramen magnum meningiomas or optic sheath meningiomas. Experts on these specialized localizations of meningiomas present their experience.

SpringerNeurosurgery

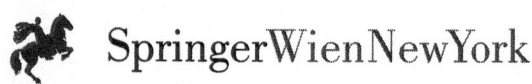

SpringerWienNewYork

P.O.Box 89, A-1201 Wien • New York, NY 10010, 175 Fifth Avenue
Heidelberger Platz 3, D-14197 Berlin • Tokyo 113, 3-13, Hongo 3-chome. Bunkyo-ku

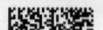